Stop Overeating and Lose Weight Easy

SECRET STRATEGIES TO BE FREE TO LOSE WEIGHT WITHOUT TAKING IT BACK AND CREATING A BETTER SELF-IMAGE

HAN CARREL

> For any communication of curiosity, possible errors or inconvenience in using the book, you can send an email to support@bookyourdestiny.com one of our consultants will respond within 48 hours.

Published by: www.bookyourdestiny.com

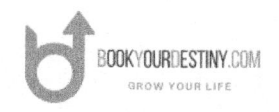

BOOKYOURDESTINY.COM
GROW YOUR LIFE

ISBN 9798387260537

First Edition: march 2023

© Copyright 2021 by Book Your Destiny - All rights reserved. The content contained within this book may not be reproduced, duplicated or transmitted without direct written permission from the author or the publisher. Under no circumstances will any blame or legal responsibility be held against the publisher, or author, for any damages, reparation, or monetary loss due to the information contained within this book; either directly or indirectly.

Cover: Book Your Destiny

All designs and pictures are property of Book Your Destiny or the source indicated

Disclaimer

Please note the information contained within this document is for educational and entertainment purposes only. All effort has been executed to present accurate, up-to-date, and reliable, complete information. No warranties of any kind are declared or implied. Readers acknowledge that the author is not engaging in the rendering of legal, financial, medical or professional advice.

ALL BOOKS OF BOOK YOUR DESTINY: www.bookyourdestiny.com

CONTENTS

CHAPTER #1 - WHAT TO WRESTLE WITH MIND OR BODY? 11

How to Work to Lose Weight (physically and psychologically) 11

How to work the eating addiction 12

What are eating disorders? 12

Bulimia nervosa... 12

Binge Eating 14

Anorexia Nervosa.. 15

Awareness 18

Overfilled tummy, less bone strength 18

The more you become obese, the less you will be able to breathe 18

Great fat leads to less fertility 19

The fat barrier in the cardiovascular system 20

Conclusion... 21

Emotional Eating Tyranny 21

Habitual overeating 21

Emotional overeating to relieve a negative emotional state 22

Overeating despite aversive consequences 22

CHAPTER #2 - HOW DOES IT WORK? 25

The connection between emotions and food 25

Impacts of Salts and Sugar on the human body 27

On Kidneys.. 27

On Heart... 29

Institutional Role 31

CHAPTER #3 - FROM SELF-DESTRUCTION TO SELF-RECONSTRUCTION 33

How you destroy yourself 33

Low energy-High addiction 34

Craving for food despite being full 35

Eating more than the real intention 36

Eat until your stomach is about to explode 36

Feeling guilty after overeating but continuing to do so 36

Making lame excuses after eating 36

Keep Failing at setting rules 37

Hiding you're eating habit from others 37

Unable to quit despite physical problems 37

Willpower and vision 38

How You Sabotage Yourself 39

It's healthy! 40

I deserve this 40

I don't want to waste food 40

I'm very tired 40

I am so stressed 40

It's so delicious 41

I might get hungry later 41

I worked so hard 41

How to Avoid Food 41

Take a walk 41

Read a book beside a window 42

Call a friend, sibling, or parents 42
Meditate... 42
Play puzzle or board games.................................... 42
Do a workout.. 42
Keep yourself hydrated 43

CHAPTER #4 - SELF-EMPOWERMENT....................44
What is Self-Empowerment? 44
Obesity and Self-empowerment 44
Relax Your Relationship with Food....................... 45
Mindless Eating.. 46
Night-time noshing... 47
Skipping Breakfast 47
Emotional Overeating 47
Eating in-Haste 48
Discover People's Value (Coaching to find out personal values that they must drive to purpose)...................... 48
  Caching Exercises 49
  Burpees 50
  Kettlebell swings 50
  Mountain climbing 51
  Renegade rows 52
  Squats 53
  The fundamental emotions for the best result 53
  How do emotions work? 54

CHAPTER #5 - DIET AND SPORTS.........................58
Are You a Smoker? Loss Weight Better 59
Diets that work 60

1. The Mediterranean Diet 61
2. The DASH Diet 62
3. Flexitarian Diet 63
4. Mediterranean-DASH Intervention for Neurodegenerative Delay Diet 64
5. Weight Watchers 66
6. Irregular Fasting 66
7. The Volumetric Diet 67

Sport Ways for Weight Loss 68
    Swimming 68
    Running 69
    Racquetball 69
    Soccer 70
    Basketball 71
    Boxing 71
    Cycling 72
    Indoors 72
    Outdoors 73

Personalize Your Best Food Plan 73

CHAPTER #6 – STRATEGIES 76
NLP Restructuring Exercise 76
Theory of NLP 77
How NLP Helps in Controlling Your Overeating Habit 78
New Body, New Life 79
Reconditioning Emotions 81
You Achieved Your Goal 83

CHAPTER #7 - TECHNIQUES TO APPLY 87

Good Foods and Bad Foods 87
Good and Bad Ways of Eating 89
Best Food Plan 90
    Step 1: Make a Menu First 90
    Step 2: Stock Your Pantry and Freezer with the Five Food Groups 92
    Step 3: Keep a Running Grocery List 94
    TELL ME ABOUT YOU 99
CONCLUSION **105**
REFERENCES **106**

INTRODUCTION

Food and weight problems and related frame photograph issues affect a huge portion of the world's population. You can be one of the over 1 billion adults worldwide (in 2008) who have been obese and more than 1/2 of one thousand million who have been considered obese (World Health Organization 2014). Even if you are not obese, you can have troulbles with meal problems, inclunding meal cravings, meal fears, or compulsive overeating. You can also have body image problems in that you experience your frame has betrayed you by no longer being in the form or in the size you'd need it to be, or for some reason , you can experience disenchanted together with your body.

If any of this is true, you will be spending a while demanding approximately your look or body size, searching for shed pounds or preventing now no longer regain the weight you've lost, attempting diets, demanding approximately purchasing for clothes, and feeling ashamed of ways you look. You can also find that dieting is not doing well—at least in the long run. If you feel hopeless or experience nothing has truly woeked for you, this book will make lots of sense. This e-book will assist you in recognizing why you have had such a hassle with your weight.

You will learn how your weight, meals, and body image problems are related to your experiences as a toddler or an adult, your emotions and ideals you've formed (generally unconsciously) approximately yourself, and lifestyles that preserve you stuck. However, except telling you the "why" of your meals and weight problems, this e-book will offer you approaches to do away with those blocks and additionally realistic and sustainable answers for the not unusual place pitfalls that maximum human beings with meals, weight, and body image problems conflict with—problems which include a way to stop emotional eating, address pressure without meals, and do away with blocks to moving your body.

Most importantly, you will discover ways to focus on your attention approximately your meals and body image problems, and your weight from an area of dissatisfaction and not anything-ever-works hopelessness to one in all attaining your desires with the aid of using dwelling to fulfill your soul, not the scale. This might also look like an overseas idea, but simply ask yourself why you need to shed pounds, why you're truly disenchanted with your frame, or why you truly overeat.

Perhaps you, like the various customers I work with who have those problems, secretly experience that if you may simply be skinny or simply shed pounds, then your lifestyles could work out. In fact, it's the alternative manner around. If you may stay with greater pleasure in your lifestyle, attaining a wholesome weight will become much less difficult. If this announcement confuses you, this book will show evidence that what I'm pronouncing truly works.

This book gathers all I've found within the past ten years—among therapy, relationships, workshops I've attended and led, retreats I've participated in, lectures I've given, letters, and phone calls. The book is a compilation of years of getting to know and suffering and loving funneled into and tailored to resolve the conflicts based on emotional consumption. Because the manner of breaking loose is a completely non-public one—all of us struggle with specific internal demons, though they take place themselves in similar styles of consuming—this book is a completely non-public one.

This is a manual for each day's support, direction, and encouragement. By imparting gear to paintings with, and on which you may elaborate, it interprets the mild philosophy of the breaking free workshops—trusting yourself, nourishing yourself, accepting yourself—into each day's moves and beliefs. Although I even have inferred all through the book that a first-rate aspect of being fat is emotional consuming, I need to strain that I now no longer agree that each human being who is obese is an emotional eater. Despite the voluminous number of studies on weight-reduction plans and being fats, we do not understand why humans who devour the same sorts and quantities of meals are available in specific sizes. It appears that it's a mixture of heredity, early metabolism, and activity levels. All heavier human beings also appear to devour greater than their lighter counterparts. Not everybody fat is an emotional eater.

Not everybody who's fats is the usage of their weight to explicit tangled emotions.

Not everybody whose fats are psychically making the most of it. Not everybody who's fats desires to be thinner. I even have written this book, due to the fact I agree with its higher to be thinner, however due to the fact I even have skilled the ache of revolving my lifestyles around meals. I'm not talking to the human beings who might be massive and dwelling absolutely that I speak; however, to the human beings who, at any weight, are using meals instead for collaborating in their lives. I hope the book will encourage you to deal with yourself and you're consumed with perception and compassion and that this perception and compassion will enlarge everybody you touch. Most of all, I want you to break free from your own.

CHAPTER #1 - WHAT TO WRESTLE WITH MIND OR BODY?

How to Work to Lose Weight (physically and psychologically)

Obesity is commonly assumed to be associated with psychological and emotional complications. Over the years, research on the psychosocial aspects of obesity has progressed from purely theoretical papers to cross-sectional comparisons of people with and without physical problems to prospective studies of the temporal sequence of obesity and mood disturbance. Obesity is not systematically associated with psychopathological outcomes in these studies. Certain obese people, on the other hand, are at a higher risk of psychiatric disorders, particularly depression [1].

You are about to lower your weight and overcome your overeating habit. Still, when food comes in front of you, you lose control and begin to eat until your stomach is about to explode due to overfilling. You are not alone in this. Many people deal with a similar problem when they are about to follow their diet plan. This is a psychological and habitual barrier between you and your thoughts about what to eat. Most people find themselves weaker in resisting food, specifically industrially processed and fast food. Recent studies have revealed a strong connection between psychological variables like emotional dysregulation, mood, health literacy, etc., and binge eating habits. They interact with the executive functioning of people, which causes people to fail to stick with their plan [2].

Obesity is a classic example of behavior whose explanation falls under psychology, economics, and the biological sciences. While psychologists and public health advocates have long viewed overeating as a flaw or disease that requires treatment, economists have pointed out that, like any other consumer behavior, diet and exercise choices can be seen through the lens of rational decision theory, subject to the influence of price and income variation but not necessarily as a problem that requires a solution [3].

How to work the eating addiction

Multiple factors are involved, which lowers the strength of people to come out of their comfort zone. Among them, an important one is that processed food is addictive. Such edibles contain many sugars, preservatives, salts, fats, etc. You might be wondering how much stuff is addictive. It's not their physical appearance; it's their chemical structural resemblance with narcotics like cocaine, opioids, and heroin. Most narcotics are addictive because they temporarily develop a sense of pleasure, and the person craves that feeling, leading to addiction [4]. For instance, high consumption of sugars produces a similar impact to cocaine. It may be due to both inducing a feeling of reward and pleasure [5].

It has a disastrous impact on your brain, which reduces your resistance toward the food and makes you eat irregularly. Intake of sugars deactivates your brain. Your brain has an essential role in regulating the intake of food. More specifically, the hypothalamus part of the brain is responsible for this regulation. The Ventral Tegmental Area of the brain regulates the sense after the ingestion. When you ingest a high number of sugars, it deactivates your brain or hypothalamus for almost 12 minutes and makes you feel good. It is also related to your satiety effect of yours. It is because sugars have to be metabolized first [6].

What are eating disorders?

In this section, I would like to talk about ailments related to your eating habits, especially if you like to eat at irregular intervals. If you are obese, you may have one or more such disorders. They are vital because they are often neglected, and the person has to deal with the consequences.

Bulimia nervosa

One of the most crucial eating disorders is bulimia nervosa. Bulimia nervosa patients alternate dieting or eating only low-calorie "safe foods" with binge eating on "forbidden" high-calorie foods. Binge eating is defined as eating a large amount of food in a short period while feeling out of control of what or how much one is eating. Binge eating is typically hidden and accompanied by feelings of shame or embarrassment. Binges can be massive, and food is frequently consumed quickly, beyond fullness, causing nausea and discomfort. Binges happen at least once a week and are usually followed by "compensatory behaviors" in order to prevent weight gain. Fasting, vomiting, laxative abuse, and compulsive exercise are the behaviors shown.

Bulimia nervosa patients, like anorexics, are excessively preoccupied with food, weight, or shape, negatively affecting and disproportionately impacting their self-worth. Individuals suffering from bulimia nervosa can be underweight, average, overweight, or obese. If they are underweight, they are diagnosed with anorexia nervosa binge-eating/purging rather than bulimia nervosa. Family members and friends may be unaware that a person suffers from bulimia nervosa because they do not appear underweight and because their behaviors are hidden and may go unnoticed by those close to them.

The signs that someone may have bulimia nervosa are:

- ✓ Frequently go to the bathroom immediately after eating.
- ✓ Loss of large amounts of food or unexplained empty packaging or food containers.
- ✓ Chronic sore throat.
- ✓ Swelling of the salivary glands on the cheeks Caries caused by gastric acid erosion of tooth enamel.
- ✓ Heartburn and gastroesophageal reflux disease Abuse of laxatives or diet pills.
- ✓ Diarrhea of unknown cause for recurrence Abuse of diuretics (drugs).
- ✓ Dizziness or fainting due to excessive urinary behavior leading to dehydration
- ✓ Bulimia nervosa can cause rare but fatal complications such as esophageal lacerations, stomach ruptures, and dangerous arrhythmias. Medical monitoring of severe bulimia nervosa is essential for identifying and treating potential complications. Outpatient cognitive-behavioral therapy for bulimia nervosa is the treatment with the most robust evidence. It helps patients deal with thoughts and emotions that normalize their diet and

perpetuate their disability. Antidepressants can also help reduce the urge to make noise and vomiting. [7]

Binge Eating

Binge-eating disorder is a severe eating disorder in which you consume large amounts of food regularly without being able to stop. On rare occasions, almost everyone overeats, such as having seconds or thirds of a holiday meal. Excessive overeating that feels out of control and becomes a habit for some people, however, crosses the line into binge-eating disorder. You may feel embarrassed about overeating if you have a binge-eating disorder and vow to stop. But you are so compelled that you cannot resist the urges and continue binge eating.

The reason for discussing binge eating is that almost all the fat guys do that in one way or another. It is sometimes confused with bulimia nervosa. However, unlike bulimia, you do not regularly compensate for extra calories eaten by vomiting, using laxatives, or exercising excessively after a binge. You can diet or eat normally. However, limiting your diet may lead to more binge eating. Most people with binge eating disorders are overweight or obese, but you could be of average weight.

The following are behavioral and emotional signs and symptoms of binge eating disorder:

- ✓ Eating huge amounts of food in a short period, such as two hours
- ✓ Feeling like you're eating habits are out of control
- ✓ Eating even if you're not hungry or full
- ✓ Rapid eating during binge episodes
- ✓ Consuming food until you are uncomfortably full
- ✓ Eating alone or in secret frequently Feeling depressed, disgusted, ashamed, guilty, or upset about your eating
- ✓ Dieting frequently, possibly without weight loss

Seek medical attention as soon as possible if you have symptoms of bulimia. Binge problems can last for years, from short-term to relapse, if left untreated. Talk to your doctor or mental health professional about the symptoms and feelings of bulimia. If you are hesitant to receive treatment, talk to someone you can trust about what you are experiencing. Friends, loved ones, teachers, or religious leaders can help you take the first steps towards successfully treating bulimia nervosa.[8]

Anorexia Nervosa

Anorexia nervosa is characterized by self-starvation and weight loss, resulting in low stature and age. Anorexia nervosa has the highest mortality rate of any psychiatric diagnosis except opioid use disorder and can be a severe condition. Body mass index (BMI, a measure of height and weight) is usually less than 18.5 in adults with anorexia nervosa. The dieting behavior of anorexia nervosa is caused by an intense fear of gaining or gaining weight. Some people with anorexia nervosa try to gain weight because they want to gain weight. Still, their behavior is not in line with that intention. For example, they may only eat small amounts of low-calorie foods and exercise excessively. Some persons with anorexia nervosa also intermittently binge eat or purge by vomiting or laxative misuse.

There are two subtypes of anorexia nervosa:

1. Restricting type, in which individuals lose weight primarily by dieting, fasting, or excessively exercising, and
2. Binge-eating/purging is when people also engage in intermittent binge eating and/or purging behaviors.

Over time, some of the following symptoms may develop related to starvation or purging behaviors:

1. Menstrual periods cease
2. Dizziness or fainting from dehydration
3. Brittle hair/nails
4. Cold intolerance

5. Muscle weakness and wasting
6. Heartburn and reflux (in those who vomit)
7. Severe constipation, bloating, and fullness after meals.
8. Stress fractures from compulsive exercise as well as bone loss resulting in osteopenia or osteoporosis (thinning of the bones)
9. Depression, irritability, anxiety, poor concentration, and fatigue

Serious medical complications can be life-threatening and include heart rhythm abnormalities, especially in those patients who vomit or use laxatives, kidney problems, or seizures. Treatment for anorexia nervosa involves helping those affected normalize their eating and weight control behaviors and restore their weight. Medical assessment and treatment of concomitant psychiatric or medical conditions are essential for treatment planning. Dietary planning should focus on helping individuals combat their anxiety about their diet and practicing a balanced diet of various foods of varying calorie densities with regularly spaced meals.

For adolescents, the most effective treatment is to help parents support and monitor their child's diet. Dealing with physical dissatisfaction is also essential, but correction often takes longer than weight and eating habits. For severe anorexia nervosa, inpatients or inpatients may be required to be admitted to a behavioral specialty program if outpatient treatment is ineffective. Most specialized programs effectively recover weight and normalize dietary patterns. Still, the risk of recurrence remains vital during the first year after discharge from the program.[9]

The risk of eating disorders varies in men and women. According to some studies, these miseries are more common in women than men. It's no surprise that most men's ideal body shape is a large, muscular body. On the contrary, women often aim to achieve a toned and lean body. Social media also has an impact on how people feel about their bodies. A study on social media use and body satisfaction observed that increased social media use tended to be associated with lower body satisfaction. Low levels of body satisfaction are also associated with higher rates of eating disorders. Cultural differences in ideal body types predispose women to eating disorders. While men tend to eat more food, women try to limit their calorie intake, which can do in very unhealthy ways [10].

The graph shows that eating disorders are more common in females than males.

Source: https://mirror-mirror.org/facts-staticstics/graphs-on-eating-disorders

To summarize this, the following table may help you to understand it better:

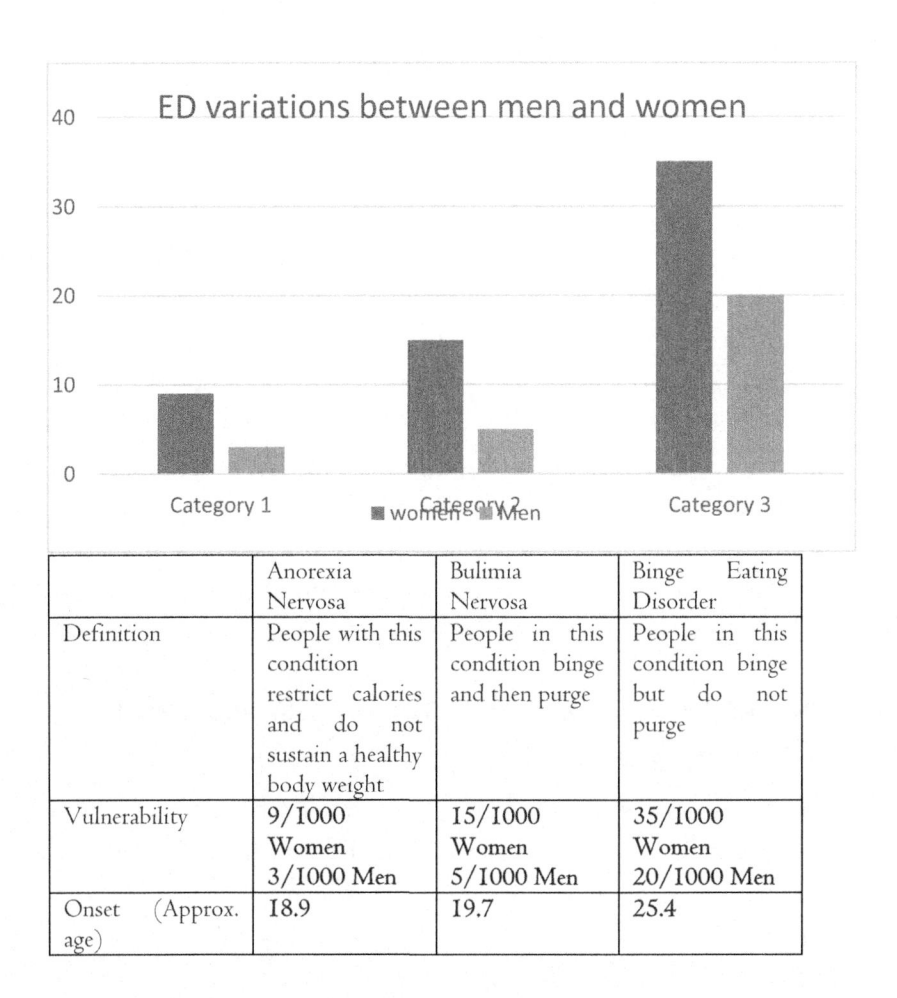

ED variations between men and women

(Bar chart showing women and men across Category 1, Category 2, Category 3)

	Anorexia Nervosa	Bulimia Nervosa	Binge Eating Disorder
Definition	People with this condition restrict calories and do not sustain a healthy body weight	People in this condition binge and then purge	People in this condition binge but do not purge
Vulnerability	9/1000 Women 3/1000 Men	15/1000 Women 5/1000 Men	35/1000 Women 20/1000 Men
Onset (Approx. age)	18.9	19.7	25.4

Awareness

Being healthy is gook, but being overweight is not. Whatever you eat may give such an experience to your taste buds which they never had before, but at what cost? What do you lose just to fulfil your urge for that food which you have never eaten before? I am going to answer these questions which may make you think about your intake habits:

Overfilled tummy, less bone strength

Recent epidemiological and animal studies data strongly support that fat accumulation is detrimental to bone mass. As far as we know, obesity can affect bone metabolism through multiple mechanisms. Because adipocytes and osteoblasts are derived from normal pluripotent mesenchymal stem cells, obesity may increase adipocyte differentiation and fat accumulation and reduce osteoblast differentiation and bone formation.

Obesity is associated with chronic inflammation. Increased circulatory and tissue pro-inflammatory cytokines in obesity can promote osteoclast activity and bone resorption by modifying NF-KB (RANK) / RANK ligand/osteoprotegerin signaling receptor activators. In addition, obese adipocyte hypersecretion and/or decreased adiponectin production directly affects bone formation or indirectly affects bone resorption through upregulated inflammatory cytokine production. Can affect. Finally, high fat intake can interfere with calcium absorption in the intestine and thus reduce the availability of calcium for bone formation. Elucidating the relationship between fat and bone metabolism at the molecular level may help design treatments to prevent or treat both obesity and osteoporosis. [11]

The more you become obese, the less you will be able to breathe

Obesity is a pandemic worldwide and increases the risk of cardiovascular disease, type 2 diabetes, and certain types of cancer. In addition, obesity is currently recognized as an essential risk factor for developing some respiratory illnesses. Of these respiratory disorders, it is already well known that obesity can lead to obstructive sleep apnea (OSA) and obesity hypoventilation syndrome (OHS). Recent data suggest that the prevalence of wheezing and bronchial hypersensitivity, two commonly associated asthma symptoms, is increased in people who are overweight or obese. In fact, epidemiological studies have reported that obesity is a risk factor for developing asthma. In addition, many studies have shown that obesity is associated with an increased risk of developing deep vein thrombosis, pulmonary embolism, pulmonary hypertension, and pneumonia. Finally, weight loss effectively improves the symptoms and severity of some respiratory symptoms, including OSA and asthma. Therefore, overweight and obese patients should be encouraged to lose weight to reduce their risk of respiratory illness or to improve the course of their existing condition.[12]

Great fat leads to less fertility

Polycystic ovary syndrome (PCOS) is one of the women's most common causes of an ovulatory infertility. The clinical characteristics of PCOS are heterogeneous and can change throughout life, from puberty to postmenopausal age. It depends primarily on obesity and metabolic changes such as insulin resistance and metabolic syndrome, which consistently affect most women with PCOS. Indeed, obesity has severe implications for both the pathophysiology and clinical manifestations of PCOS.

This is because various mechanisms lead to hyperandrogenism, excess and increased availability of free androgens, and changes in granulosa cell function and follicular development. Notably, simple obesity itself represents a functional high androgenic state. These mechanisms include early hormone and metabolic factors during intrauterine life, leptin, insulin, the insulin growth factor system, and possibly the endogenous cannabinoid system.

Compared to normal-weight women with PCOS, obese women are characterized by poor androgen and metabolic status, poor menstrual and ovulatory performance, and ultimately reduced pregnancy rates. The importance of obesity in the etiology of PCOS is highlighted by metabolic changes and the effectiveness of lifestyle interventions and weight loss on hyperandrogenism, ovulation, and fertility. The increased prevalence of obesity in adolescents and young women with PCOS may be partially associated with an increasing epidemic of obesity worldwide. Still, this hypothesis is supported by long-term prospective epidemiological studies.[13]

In the case of men, several studies show that obese men are more likely to have abnormal semen parameters and that a couple whose male partner is overweight is at increased risk of infertility. Therefore, obesity is associated with a high incidence of male infertility. Many mechanisms are responsible for the effects of obesity on male infertility by inducing sleep apnea, altered hormonal profiles (decreased active in B and androgen levels with elevated estrogen levels), and elevated scrotal temperatures. This appears as a disorder of semen (total sperm count, concentration, decreased motility, increased DNA fragmentation index). However, neither the reversibility of obesity-related male infertility with weight loss nor effective therapeutic interventions have been extensively studied. Increasing the prevalence of obesity requires greater clinical awareness of its effects on fertility, a better understanding of the underlying mechanisms, and an investigation of treatment routes.[14]

The fat barrier in the cardiovascular system

Obesity is a significant granter widespread cardiovascular disease in underdeveloped and developed worlds. Obesity is a chronic metabolic disorder associated with many heart diseases and increased morbidity. Many adaptations/alterations in cardiac structure and function occur as excess adipose tissue accumulates, even without comorbidities. Alternation from high physical to less demanding life can be observed today throughout several nations.

This misfortune associated with obesity implicates a corresponding increase in the number of individuals afflicted with metabolic syndrome, which defines the obese patient as "at stake." Adipose tissue is not simply a passive storage site for fat but an endocrine organ capable of synthesizing and releasing into the bloodstream various molecules that may impact the risk unfavorably for the obese. Indeed, obesity may affect atherosclerosis through unknown variables and risk factors for coronary artery disease such as dyslipidemia, hypertension, glucose intolerance, inflammatory markers, and the prothrombotic state. Therefore, doctors usually recommend weight loss to treat heart diseases. [15]

Conclusion

Here you read some of the major disasters caused by high-fat accumulation in the body. If the person lacks physical activities like exercise, walking, etc., it fuels the fire. Moreover, irregular pattern of eating and especially binge eating fills the remaining vacant space. In this way, it causes damage to your health and makes you a victim of body-shaming. You usually read this quote, especially on roads.

"Smokers die young."

This is valid for smokers and those who overeat processed and fast food. Because overeaters and obese are at greater risk of developing numerous heart and other diseases. So now, whether you want to stop binge eating and start losing weight or keep living in your comfort zone, it's in your hands.

Emotional Eating Tyranny

Many people develop excessive eating habits due to emotional causes. Food, especially processed and fast food, induces a sense of pleasure because it contains ingredients that chemically resemble addictive drugs. So, people tend to eat, especially, sweet food like ice cream, chocolates, etc.

Below there are three main reasons which cause emotional eating?

1. Habitual overeating
2. Overeating to relieve a negative emotional state
3. Overeating despite aversive consequences [16]

Habitual overeating

To be considered an overeating addict, they must eat large amounts of food, whether hungry or not. This can manifest itself in different ways. Some people can eat large amounts of food at once. Someone struggling with compulsive overeating may also graze each other. Grazing is when someone sips continuously throughout the day, even when they're not hungry [17]

However, people who force overeating may use food as the only means of dealing with negative emotions. As a result, they often feel that their eating is out of control. They think about food and feel guilty, ashamed, or depressed after eating. It's very different from how one feels after eating a hearty Thanksgiving meal. You may feel full and regret eating that last piece of cake, but you don't have to gnaw at it out of shame [18].

Emotional overeating to relieve a negative emotional state

The emotional eating theory states that negative emotions promote eating because eating is likely to reduce intensity. Emotional eating is thought to be reasonably expected. Still, individuals vary significantly in how much food they consume to improve their mood. The cause of these differences is unknown, and there is no clear evidence for the origin of this type of diet. Theories point to a connection between influences and food in childhood, but cultural influences later in life and certain biological factors (e.g., sensitivity to taste) may also play some role.

We know a little more about the underlying mechanics. When ingested, foods can induce robust hedonic responses that enhance emotional states. Once ingested, nutrients can influence the neurochemical and endocrine systems involved in emotions. The activation of these psychological (pleasure) and physiological (neurochemical) mechanisms may depend on the extent of emotional eating. Allergic reactions are likely to occur in most cases of emotional eating. Still, a certain amount of energy-rich food is required to exert the neurochemical and neuroendocrine effects [19].

Overeating despite aversive consequences

Loss of control over food and drug-seeking and using behaviors is considered an intractable aspect of addiction, leading to constant use despite the many negative consequences that lead to repressive behaviors. Regime. However, despite the many negative consequences caused by such behavior, it is still challenging for individuals to stop. "Losing control" results from a deficit in the inhibitory control mechanisms responsible for preventing inappropriate actions. These deficits can lead to vulnerability to addictive behavior and/or result from persistent and prolonged drug use or overconsumption of palatable foods.

People with compulsive eating disorders show poor performance in food-related executive function and inhibitory control tasks, such as response restriction, appetite suppression, or delayed refreshments. These deficiencies are associated with additional weight gain and a poorer response to weight loss treatment. This loss of control over overeating often persists despite many adverse events, including physical, psychological, and social problems that arise or are aggravated by overeating. In fact, compulsive overeating often struggles with overeating, citing reactions of shame, denial, rationalization, blame, and a sense of loss of control. When these negative mental and physical consequences outweigh the desired effects of palatable foods, people often attempt to diet and avoid the triggering foods, although most relapse into eating habits. Unhealthy drinking.

Within this theoretical framework, compulsion-like behavior is operated in preclinical research as seeking reward despite adverse conditions or consequences. Some models have suggested that compulsive eating behaviors may become apparent after a history of eating palatable foods. For example, animals exhibit compulsive behavior, such as consuming delicious food with a mild electric shock or a conditioned stimulus signaling an electric shock. Animals will also continue to eat palatable foods even if they are subjected to an unpleasant condition (i.e., overcoming a new, bright, and potentially dangerous environment to obtain that food) or comply with a progressive rate process where the reaction cost increases with each reward. [20]

These psychological and emotional aspects clearly show that the biggest hurdle in overcoming eating habits and losing weight is highly dependent on your psychological and emotional control over yourself. One can possibly control compulsive eating only if one can overpower one's mind. At the onset of their execution of the plan, most people are very excited and enthusiastic. Still, as time proceeds, they lose heart just because they cannot see a visible change in them. Always remember one thing that good things take time to happen. It requires a lot of patience and continuous work. All you have to do is stick with your diet plan and daily workout. You will be able to see the change in yourself sooner or later, but you will.

CHAPTER #2 - HOW DOES IT WORK?

"I overcame my psychological barrier. What's next?" You may encounter this question when you decide to leave all your bad habits and desire to make your ideal body type. Men prefer a big muscular body while women go for a thin body with a tiny waist. It has been found that people focus more on their workouts than their diet. They presume that a workout is the only way to get what they want. At the same time, in the case of diet, they usually think eating less and exercising more would be beneficial.

The measurement of weight-loss diets is an important unresolved issue; current dietary patterns, regular diets, desire to lose weight, specific weight control behaviors, and weight changes may have different health effects and require to be distinguished; weight-loss diets are not generally associated with nutritional deficiencies, adverse physiological adaptations, severe psychological reactions, or the development of eating disorders; and recommendations against weight loss efforts involving moderate changes in diet and exercise routine are not warranted [21]. This chapter will describe how to work to get your ideal body. We shall also focus on those workouts and diet plans, which will act as a catalyst in its persuasion. Moreover, we shall also talk about what emotions you should have to fulfil your mission.

The connection between emotions and food

Emotions and food and drink consumption are inextricably linked. As sensory and consumer science seeks to conceptualize the consumer experience better, there is growing interest in measuring emotions. Emotions can provide critical information for distinguishing products, predicting consumer choices, and providing details about product perceptions. Several emotion measurement tools include physiological methods, face recognition, and self-reported verbal and visual emotion measurement [22].

It was described in the previous chapter that people develop their eating habits in order to alter their negative moods. Because processed food contains items that resemble chemically addictive drugs, there are several ways by which food can drive your neurons. This way, you would go against your plan of becoming intelligent and muscular. The relationship between diet and mental health is complicated. But research shows a tie between what we eat and how we feel. If you eat well, you will feel better.

You don't have to make significant changes to your diet, but see if you can try some of these tips:

- ✓ Eat regularly. It will prevent your blood sugar from dropping, and you may feel tired or moody.

- ✓ Keep yourself hydrated because even mild dehydration can affect your mood, energy levels, and concentration.

- ✓ Eat the right balance of fat. Your brain needs healthy fats to function well. They are found in olive oil, canola oil, nuts, seeds, oily fish, avocados, milk, eggs, etc.

- ✓ Avoid Tran's fats, common in processed and packaged foods, as they can adversely affect mood and heart health.

- ✓ Incorporate more whole grains, fruits, and vegetables into your diet. They contain the vitamins and minerals your brain and body need to stay healthy.

- ✓ Add protein to every diet. It contains amino acids that your brain uses to regulate your mood.

- ✓ Take care of your intestinal health. Your gut can reflect how you feel: it can speed up or slow down when stressed.

- ✓ A healthy intestinal diet includes fruits, vegetables, beans, and probiotics. Be aware of how caffeine affects your mood.

- ✓ Drinking before bedtime can cause some people to have sleep problems, frustration and anxiety. Caffeine is found in coffee, tea, cola, energy drinks, and chocolate [23]

Impacts of Salts and Sugar on the human body

Before moving further, I have a question for you: Have you ever eaten from palatable food brands like McDonald's or KFC? If the answer is yes, then even after eating, you urged for more, and you want to eat it daily? Have you ever noticed that secret ingredient makes you crave it? The answer to all of these questions is there is no secret ingredient but salts, sugars and fats. Together or separately, they induce the production of dopamine, a brain chemical responsible for the feelings of pleasure and reward.

> **Do you know?**
>
> **Your daily salt requirement is 2300 mg. However, 9 nuggets of McDonald's without sauce contain 0.77 g of salt.**

It gives your taste buds such a marvelous experience but damages your inner health. Salt is an essential compound for our health. However, if it is too much, it can adversely affect the body's ability to function properly. Table salt is actually sodium chloride. It is a mineral widely distributed in nature and the human body. Unfortunately, most people consume excessive salt – about 3.4g per day. This is more than twice the required intake. Excessive sodium intake over such a long period causes many complications, especially for the kidneys. The kidneys have difficulty removing excess salt and water from the blood. The kidney is considered an important organ. They are responsible for filtering your blood to remove toxins and excess water. Their function is to maintain the balance of water, salt and minerals in the blood [24]

On Kidneys

Over-intake of salts leads to high blood pressure and kidney disease. High blood pressure puts extra pressure on the kidney's filtration unit and can lead to scarring. This impairs the kidneys' ability to regulate water and raises blood pressure. "If you don't stop this cycle, it can lead to kidney disease and kidney failure," said Dr George Thomas, a hypertension specialist director of the Center for Blood Pressure Disorders in the Kidney and Hypertension

Department. "High blood pressure and uncontrolled diabetes are the most common causes of kidney disease."

Unfortunately, most people, with kidney disease, are unaware of that. Signs and symptoms can be due to other medical conditions and usually appear when the kidneys have already begun to malfunction.

The symptoms to watch out for are:

- ✓ Abnormal fatigue.
- ✓ Sleep disorders.
- ✓ Itchy skin.
- ✓ Reduced urination.
- ✓ Blood or bubbles in the urine.
- ✓ Swelling around the ankles, feet, or eyes.
- ✓ Loss of appetite, nausea, or vomiting.
- ✓ Muscle cramps.
- ✓ Abnormal taste. [25]

Consult your doctor if you have any of these symptoms, especially if you are over 60 years old and are at risk of kidney disease due to a family history of high blood pressure, diabetes, or kidney failure. Kidney health and salt intake.

> **Do you know?**
>
> **The two kidneys purify approximately 180 liters of blood.**

Sugar is not a problem for your kidneys unless your blood sugar is too high. This is common in both type 1 and types 2 diabetes. As soon as the blood sugar level exceeds 180 mg/dl, the kidneys release sugar into the urine. The higher the blood sugar level, the more sugar is excreted in the urine. If your kidneys are normal, this is usually not a problem. Still, if you have diabetes, too much sugar can damage your kidneys. Unchecked diabetes can damage the blood vessels in the kidneys and destroy the filters. At this point, the kidneys can no longer work effectively. When the blood vessels in the kidneys are damaged, the kidneys cannot purify the blood properly, retain more water and salt, and waste products accumulate in the blood [26]

> **Do you know?**
>
> **The normal amount of sugar in the blood is 180 mg/dl**

On Heart

In modern medicine, people tend to have negative feelings about sodium, an element contained in salt. Too high sodium intake is associated with water retention and hypertension risk factor. Excessive sodium intake and hypertension develop heart failure and major risk factors for complications in patients with existing heart failure. As 6.5 million American adults suffer from heart failure, limiting salt intake can significantly reduce the risk of this major medical tragedy. Sodium intake is associated with fluid retention, so there is swelling and bloating that follows a very salty diet. And excessive sodium intake can exacerbate high blood pressure or high blood pressure.

High blood pressure increases the risk of developing heart failure and exacerbates existing heart failure. High blood pressure can cause other heart diseases, stroke, or kidney failure. A low-salt diet helps reduce or prevent high blood pressure and may reduce the risk of such illness. This kind of diet is usually high in total fat and calories and can cause obesity and many associated complications. Some studies suggest sodium intake may be associated with osteoporosis and gastric cancer. In addition, long-term eating of salty foods can help the taste buds become accustomed to the taste buds, which in turn increases the likelihood of eating salty foods [27]

In the American diet, the main sources are soft drinks, fruit drinks, flavored yoghurt, cereals, cookies, cakes, candies, and most processed foods. However, adding sugar is also found in foods that do not seem sweet, such as soups, bread, salted meats, and ketchup. According to the National Cancer Institute, adult men consume 24 additional cups of sugar per day. That's 384 calories. According to Doctor Hu, JAMA Internal Medicine

"Basically, the higher the intake of added sugar, the higher the risk for heart disease,"

Excessive sugar intake can increase blood pressure and increase chronic inflammation. Both of these are pathological routes to heart disease. Liquid calories are not as satisfying as solid food calories, so excessive sugar intake, especially with sweet drinks, can lead to weight gain by tricking the body into turning off the appetite control system. For this reason, people find adding calories to their regular diet easier when drinking sweet drinks. [28]

> **Do you know?**
> **Our body needs 30g of sugar daily to function properly.**

One can easily assume how these brands, just for some profit, put your health in danger. The daily requirement of your salt and sugar can easily be obtained but consuming junk food increases the sugar and salt level in the body to a disastrous level. Their business simply runs on one principle, "The sicker they are, the more profit we gain". They attract you by different means like their packaging, the odor of their food, its physical appearance and the list.

Some of the tricks they use to attract customers are summarized below.

- ✓ By TV ads, billboard posters, etc.
- ✓ Usually, it opens near public points like malls, parks etc., so they could get more attention.
- ✓ Food odor is a major factor that attracts you to them. it is also accompanied by the tactic of opening franchises near public places
- ✓ Limited offers and products, so they inflate demands
- ✓ They introduce combos like a hamburger with a regular drink with cheese fries. The add-ons like sauces, salad, and cheese also play a major role in lightening your emotional drive
- ✓ Brands like McDonald's also give toys with their meals. In this way, they get attraction by kids and thus, making their parents buy them the food
- ✓ Their menu is well designed by expert graphic designers who not only catch your attention but also increase your appetite [29]

Institutional Role

You will see the government introducing many policies regarding public health. Still, all of them focus on making people reduce their eating habits. Their policies usually do not involve checking these restaurants to control salt and sugar levels. It's because fast food restaurants are big businesses in the US. The figures from 2012 show over 120,000 franchised limited-service restaurants, employing about 2.6 million people. These restaurants have around $130 billion, which means approximately $400 yearly sales for each US citizen [30]. Obviously, why would our institutions take any actions against them?

Moreover, it is estimated that the fast-food industry, by 2027, will have a market of $931.7 billion, and almost 50 million people eat fast food daily, and the number is rising gradually [31]. Due to the growing market of this industry, it is estimated that only in the USA will 49.2% of people be obese [32]. That is alarming, but government and institutions are just a silent audience on it. In fact, our presidents promote the eating of fast food.

Those who pay more attention to media coverage of these Presidents' diets are more likely to consider fast food a socially acceptable diet. The craving for fast food of former US President Donald Trump is clear to everyone. Still, researchers say Trump wasn't the first president to talk about his eating habits. Former President Bill Clinton also had four bypass surgeries in 2004 and tended to prefer fast food before becoming vegan. Former President Barack Obama and First Lady Michelle Obama promoted a healthy diet. They planted vegetable fields on the grounds of the White House. However, the fast-food eating habits of Donald Trump could reverse this whole struggle [33].

The palatable food market is growing without any check. The brands continuously add addictive ingredients to their meals, making people crave them. The increase in the consumption of palatable food is alarming. In the future, we will face obesity, heart diseases and diabetes as epidemics. A review of fast food and heart health studies found that eating fast food at least once a week increased the risk of obesity, and eating fast food at least twice a week increased the risk of metabolic syndrome.

Death from diabetes and coronary artery disease. It won't increase pressure on our health department but also lowers our lifestyle. It's up to us how we resolve this issue. We need to help ourselves, and it is necessary to control our eating habits by ourselves. I will discuss how to control ourselves in upcoming chapters. Here are a few that go on a walk if you feel a little hungry. When you return, you will notice an increase in your appetite, and the food will be healthier and more delicious. Moreover, keep yourself hydrated and ensure you only eat when starving.

CHAPTER #3 - FROM SELF-DESTRUCTION TO SELF-RECONSTRUCTION

How you destroy yourself

Have you ever worked towards an important goal that would make you fail just because you did something stupid? Or you may feel stressed or anxious when trying to accomplish very important things. It makes you more frustrated, discouraged, and angry with yourself. These emotions trap you and prevent you from doing what you need to do. These are all signs of self-disturbance. Self-jamming undermines your self-confidence and self-esteem and affects your relationships with others.

Every time you try to do what you want and fail, you *"prove"* to yourself that you can't or shouldn't do it. Sabotage is often the act of secretly destroying or weakening something. It usually means the direct and intentional involvement of sabotage operatives. Therefore, the term is most commonly used in espionage and in business situations where insiders are causing damage. The term self-destruction is used when this destructive behavior is directed at you. At first, you may not realize what you are doing. But when negative habits always undermine your efforts, they can be seen as a form of psychological self-harm [34]

The same goes when you are dieting and losing weight. You work so hard on your diet and work out 5 or 6 days a week. You get close to getting your ideal weight, and then "something" happens... you go back to your old eating habits. You start saying things like, *"I'm fine during the day, but I start grazing and picking at night, then I tell myself I'll do it again tomorrow. Or, "I had a bad day eating; maybe quit smoking."* For some people, the old eating behavior can quickly return; for others, it is a slow and gradual reappearance. Then you feel so frustrated with not being able to lose weight again, and you decide to give up.

What about those situations when your diet is going well, and you're losing weight, and instead of giving you flowers for your birthday (or any other holiday), your partner gives you a box of your favorite chocolates. People who tempt you with food choices know you're avoiding them while making comments like "*One bite won't hurt you*" or "*You've come this far; you deserve only a bite.*" "*I did it, you have to try it.*" or "*It's your birthday, you must have a cake!*" Sound familiar? If so, you're not alone. Thousands of dieters suffer from similar patterns. In my experience, I often have people asking, "*Why is this happening?*" *Why can't I lose weight and keep it off? Or, "It's like I have two minds…one wants to lose weight, and the other doesn't let me." I also often hear, "Why can't my spouse (other people, friends, family members, etc.) support my weight loss efforts?*" "It's almost like everyone is trying to get me to eat and stay fat!" The answer to all these questions is the same. The **SELF-SABOTAGE**. Yes! It's you who are destroying yourself. Because you easily get attracted to food. I gave a brief introduction to food addiction in chapter I. Let me explain it a little bit more now.

Low energy-High addiction

The idea that a person can become addicted to food has recently gained importance. It comes from brain imaging and other studies on the effects of compulsive overeating on pleasure centers in the brain. Animal and human experiments show that for some people, the same reward and pleasure centers in the brain that are activated by addictive drugs such as cocaine and heroin are also activated by food, especially palatable food like

- ✓ Sugar
- ✓ Fat
- ✓ Salt

Like addictive drugs, very palatable foods trigger feel-good brain chemicals like dopamine. Once people experience the pleasure associated with increased dopamine transmission in the brain's reward pathways when eating certain foods, they quickly feel the urge to eat again. The reward cues from highly pleasurable foods can override other signals of satiety and satisfaction. As a result, people continue to eat, even when they are not hungry. Compulsive overeating is a type of behavioral addiction, which means that a person may become preoccupied with behaviors (such as eating, gambling, or shopping) that cause intense pleasure. Food addicts lose control of their eating behavior and spend too much time overeating or anticipating the emotional effects of compulsive overeating. People who show signs of food addiction can also develop a tolerance to food. They eat increasingly more, only to find that food satisfies them less.[35]

Let's talk about some symptoms which you can easily observe in yourself.

These symptoms will show you whether you are a food addict or not.

- ✓ Craving for food despite being full
- ✓ Eating more than intention
- ✓ Eating until your stomach is about to explode
- ✓ Feeling guilty after overeating but continues to do so
- ✓ Making lame excuses
- ✓ Failure to set rules
- ✓ Hiding eating from others
- ✓ Unable to quit despite physical problems

Let's discuss every symptom one by one

Craving for food despite being full

It is not uncommon to experience thirst even after eating a nutritious meal. For example, after a steak, potato, or vegetable supper, some people want ice cream for dessert. Craving and hunger are not the same. Crave occurs when you feel the urge to eat something after eating or when you are full. It is fairly common and does not necessarily mean that someone has an eating disorder.

Most people are hungry. However, if the thirst for food is frequent and difficult to satisfy or ignore, this could indicate something else. Craving is very common. Craving alone does not indicate food addiction, but it may indicate a problem if frequent cravings are difficult to ignore or satisfy. These thirsts are not about the need for energy or nutrients. The brain seeks to release dopamine, a chemical in the brain that plays a role in how people experience joy. People who show signs of bulimia may also develop certain food tolerances. They eat more and more but find more and more food full [36]

Eating more than the real intention

A single bite does not matter for some people, but when they begin to eat, a single bite turns into 10 or 20, a single slice of pizza into half of it, etc. It's like people decide that they will eat a little to control their diet, but due to their addiction or forced by colleagues, they eat more than they want.

Eat until your stomach is about to explode

"I've eaten so much that I'm about to burst!" Someone at the Thanksgiving table will probably say this version tomorrow after you stuff all your faces with turkey, mashed potatoes, sweet potatoes, and more. But how much do you need to eat for your stomach to rupture? Is that possible? *"Interestingly, if you eat too much, your stomach can rupture,"* he says. Rachel Vreeman, co-author of *"Don't Cross Eyes ... They Get Stuck That Way!"* And Associate Professor of Pediatrics, Indiana University School of Medicine. *"It's possible, but it's very rare."* [37]

> **Do you know?**
>
> **Normally, your stomach can hold about one or a half liter and does an OK job handling 3 liters of fluid. Studies show that the stomach ruptured when people tried to accommodate 5 liters of food.**

Feeling guilty after overeating but continuing to do so

Extensive eating makes you regret it. It is a sort of psychological issue related to binge eating habits. As I discussed in the above chapters, binge eating makes you regret eating an enormous amount of food but does not let you quit this habit of yours. It leads to serious psychological disorders like anxiety, depression, stress, etc. [38]

Making lame excuses after eating

The brain can be strange, especially when it comes to addiction. Choosing to move away from the trigger hood can lead someone to create your own rules. However, it can be difficult to follow these rules. When faced with cravings, overeating people may find ways to circumvent the rules and pamper their cravings. This idea may be similar to that of someone who is trying to quit smoking. This person may think he is not a smoker unless he buys a pack of cigarettes himself. Still, they were able to smoke from a friend's pack. With bulimia, it's common to set rules about eating habits and make excuses for why it's okay to break them.

Keep Failing at setting rules

When you are on a diet, you set some rules like "I won't eat fatty food" or "no fast food from today." But as the food shows up, you lose control and start eating without considering your plan. It's, again, a failure of your vision and willpower to do something or attain something you wanted desperately.

Hiding you're eating habit from others

When you eat unaccountably, you begin to hide from others. You prefer to eat alone, whether in a car, at night when everyone has gone to bed, etc.; it is fairly common in those people who are challenging their overeating but break their restrictions on them.

Unable to quit despite physical problems

The food you eat can have a significant impact on your health. In the short term, junk food can cause weight gain, acne, bad breath, malaise, poor dental health, and other common problems. Lifelong junk food intake can lead to obesity, type 2 diabetes, heart disease, Alzheimer's disease, dementia, and even some cancers. If you have any of these problems related to eating unhealthy foods but can't change your habits, you probably need help. A treatment plan developed by a qualified professional is usually recommended to overcome eating disorders.

As I said in the first chapter, whatever you are trying to do, the biggest hurdle in your way is you. Yes! Your mind lives in a comfort zone and does not want to get out. But to overcome this problem, two things should be explained: willpower and vision. What are they, and how do they play their part in controlling you're eating disorders and obesity? It shall be discussed in the next section.

Willpower and vision

Willpower has returned to contemporary psychology, drawing from conventional discourse, but the state of voluntarism in psychology remains unresolved. Will has many different meanings: self-control, determination, and effort; test the limits of endurance; the ability to influence and lead others; a visible mark of character; a measurable characteristic; an educational and training goal. Will is questioned, subordinated to other characteristics, and denied existence. Two conclusions emerge: qualitative research will enrich our understanding of will, and the history of will is essential to the understanding of psychology, showing that will is a category relevant to societies, where individual efforts, regardless of circumstances [39]

Let me ask you a simple question. Why do you want to lose weight? Is it because of some numbers of scale? Like most people, you will probably want to lose weight because you find it easier to live the life you want to live. Specifically, what that means varies from person to person. It may involve the solution or prevention of medical problems. Live to see children and grandchildren grow up. You can do activities that you enjoy (or need to), look in the mirror, or go out in public without feeling like a runaway from a circus sideshow. But whatever your real goals are, losing weight is the only thing that helps you reach those goals. It's not the ultimate goal, and it's important when working on your weight loss. To stay motivated for long-term projects like weight loss, you need to visualize the real reason for your hard work. So, let me give you a simple suggestion about what our vision should do in your quest to lose weight:

- ✓ Your vision should tell you why you need to lose weight. Why is the effort and effort to reach your goals worth it? Your answer to these *"why"* questions include some *"general"* elements (feeling comfortable, being there for grandchildren, being a good role model, the careers and relationships you want. It may contain (such as having), but as much as possible, the big picture drawn here should contain specific details. You can generate this detail by asking the following question:
- ✓ What will my life look like (1, 5, or 10) years from now? Explain what you want to do, what role you want to play, how you want to see yourself, etc.

- ✓ What are my ideal days? Explain why you are looking forward to waking up in the morning, what you do every day, who you spend with, what good experiences you want to have every day, and how you face challenges in your daily life
- ✓ What are your values (love, relationships, safety, independence, comfort, diversity, interests, enthusiasm, social contributions, family, professional success, etc.)? Do I need to express and reflect on my daily life?
- ✓ If you always need to choose from these values, please indicate how to rank these values. The vision statement does not have to include all these questions and answers. Push only key goals and concerns up. Questions are just a tool to get you thinking. You also need to include your beliefs about why it is important to lose weight to reach your *"big goals."*

The second thing a vision does give you a direction, not only towards losing weight, but your vision statement should tell you what else you need to change in your life (besides your weight) to help you go from where you are to where you are you want to be. Is. For example, you can get the list of rank values created above and compare them with those that currently seem to lead your life.

Now you can compare the perfect day with a normal day. It is important not to get angry with the current situation. Focus on what you can do to change your life in a way that suits you. If you're not ready to give up on self-blame, skip this part of your vision statement for now. Your vision statement must be in writing. It's also good to include photos and other objects to remind you of your goals and visions for difficult days. Use your vision statement regularly to remember why you're working on a weight loss plan on a particularly tough day [40]. Keep in mind that your vision is more important than your willpower. Willpower is temporary, but if your goal turns into a mission, you will be able to achieve it no matter how much fat has been accumulated in your body.

How You Sabotage Yourself

The worse thing which arrives in your quest is those lame excuses and foul justifications you give yourself when food shows up. Let's move towards those lies you tell yourself and eventually rebel against yourself.

It's healthy!

I've gained a lot of weight because I ate too much healthy food. Eating food when you're not hungry is still overeating, no matter how nutritious is the food you've eaten. If your body doesn't need those calories now, they will be stored as fat, and too much body fat is not healthy! So, you can stop making fun of it.

I deserve this

What exactly do you deserve? Do you gain weight by eating food when you are not hungry? Your body deserves to work hard for you all day long and be treated with respect and care. There are many other ways to do good for yourself without eating when you are not hungry. You can find some ideas here or create your list to use when you feel the urge to eat in the future but aren't hungry.

I don't want to waste food

Oh, an excuse for *"human trash"!* Shouldn't the extra food be wasted somehow and should be thrown into the right jar instead of being physically disposed of? Like all foods your body doesn't need, your foods to avoid waste are stored as fat. Is that what you want? Children who are hungry somewhere in the world will not benefit from eating it. It's much better to throw it away, give it as a gift, or save it for later use.

I'm very tired

Do you think you're really tired because you're not hungry but need food? Unless you are malnourished, eating does not reduce your fatigue; it increases your tiredness. Take a break and do something which makes you relax if needed.

I am so stressed

I emphasize one of my old personal favorites. Yes, food can temporarily relieve your stress, but most of the time, only when it is in your mouth. If you eat under stress, weight gain causes long-term stress and affects your physical and mental health. You may not be able to get rid of what you are feeling stressed about, but you can certainly prevent secondary stress, which is a by-product of eating as a pacifier. Going for a deep breath, meditation, or walking is just one food-free stress relief option. Try one of those and see whether your urge to eat doesn't go away.

It's so delicious
Food, no doubt, tastes good and can fill your mouth with water. But food becomes a lot tasty when you are starving. So, why not eat when you are hungry.

I might get hungry later
Preventive diet. Some examples justify eating because you don't have a chance when you're hungry, but they are rare and almost always avoided. You can carry around portable meals such as snacks and packs, so you can eat something when you start to growl. It helps you avoid being hungry enough to be less enthusiastic about what to eat later. But think about it. How often do you use it as an excuse instead of needing it?

I worked so hard
You have worked so hard changing your diet to lose weight, and now using this as an excuse to disturb yourself? Rewarding yourself with food should learn exactly what you shouldn't do. If you want to reward yourself, don't use food. It's great to reward yourself in other ways. Make a list of ways to reward yourself without eating when you're not hungry.[41]

Just think about the excuses which I discussed. How many times have you done that? These are those justifications you give yourself while you are disrupting the whole you have done for it. Whenever you want to eat but you're not hungry, stop and see what excuses you make for yourself. Next, consider whether that is true. By not making excuses for eating when you are not hungry, you will be able to take care of yourself.

How to Avoid Food
If there are several ways which can make you eat, then there are also some ways that can help you to stop thinking about food. It sounds hard but trusts me, it's really helpful to overcome your overeating habit. Let's have a look at these.

Take a walk
Get out of the kitchen, take a walk (or jogging) outside and focus on things other than food. *"The movement has also helped reduce thirst,"* said Josh York, founder and **CEO of GYMGUYZ**. *"Walking and jogging can help distract and entertain, as hunger can be caused by boredom."* *"Sometimes your body craves*

a little exercise," says nutritionist Katie. Boyd says, *"When I'm hungry, I tie my shoes and walk for about 20 minutes. When I get home, I'm completely hungry."* [42]

Read a book beside a window
Changing scenery helps you to get some time to think apart from food. The best way is to read a book you always wanted to read beside a window.

Call a friend, sibling, or parents
Call them! Pick up your phone and call someone you trust before those negative thoughts grow. It is a great opportunity to meet with your loved ones. Give them a call! Take a bubble bath or apply a face mask. *"When it comes to fascinating a treat, you can do something amazing by giving yourself time to thank your physical vessel,"* says Boyd.[43]

Meditate
Meditation teaches you to sit emotionally and observe without judgment, rather than relying on coping mechanisms such as overeating. Meditation helps us eat more carefully and even addresses emotional dietary problems that may persist [44]

Play puzzle or board games
Puzzle and board games are great for taking your attention away from food. Such games require a lot of focus, and psychologically you do it. As it may sound traditional, solving jigsaw puzzles is an easy way to spend time and can silence your mind, so you have to stop thinking about food. And if you're stuck at home with others, play some of your favorite board games. And if you are playing it with your friends or family, it gets interesting, and you get a great way to pass your time.

Do a workout
"Not only will you burn off some of the calories you might be consuming, but by staying active, your mind isn't idle, so there's less of a chance for a bored mind to convince you that you're hungry. When there isn't. Not," says **Susan E. Wilson, RDN, LDN.** *"Also, regular physical activity also helps with stress, anxiety and depression, and I think a lot of people can use it now."* [45]

Keep yourself hydrated

By drinking more water during the day, you'll keep your stomach fuller and feel less hungry. Dehydration can also translate into hunger, making you crave snacks. If you're hungry but you ate not long ago, try drinking a glass of water. If you feel like you're not drinking enough water throughout the day, you can easily figure out how many ounces you need by dividing your body weight by two.

You probably know that food attracts you in many ways, by its color, its odor, and most important of all, its taste. It's up to you how you control yourself. Self-control is everything while you are dieting and, on a quest, to lose weight. Before taking any step further, you should have a vision that won't only inspire you to do something but will also provide you with a direction. You must possess strong willpower because you can be distracted easily from it. Stay focused and work harder, and one day you will have your desired figure.

CHAPTER #4 - SELF-EMPOWERMENT

What is Self-Empowerment?

Suppose you're thinking of going back to school, applying for a promotion, or making another difference in your life. In that case, the first step is developing and accepting the confidence you need to assert yourself. Confidence doesn't just help you understand where the starting line is. It helps to set the path you take to reach your goal. Here we are, self-development is effective. A smiling student on campus. Empowered people control their lives by setting goals and taking actionable steps to achieve them. They understand how to get things done; they are confident, focused, and comfortable making decisions that will lead them to the future. If you're feeling less confident or unsure if you can achieve your ambitions, there are a few steps you can take to enjoy your life more confidently.

Self-development means making a conscious decision to take charge of your destiny. It's about making positive decisions, taking action to move forward, making decisions, and being confident in your ability in order to carry them out. Self-development people know their strengths and weaknesses and are motivated to learn and achieve them. For example, if someone is fired, they are reluctant to find a job and can wait for recruiters to find them on LinkedIn. Alternatively, you can take proactive steps to find a new and better job, such as contacting a former colleague, looking for an opportunity, or updating. Revisions of their marketable skills and their resumes. Self-development allows individuals to recognize that they have the power to make decisions that help them achieve their goals.[46]

Obesity and Self-empowerment

Obesity and low self-esteem are often closely linked. It's easy to see that overweight people suffer from self-esteem, from dealing with the judgments and comments of others to losing weight in one failed attempt at a time. Many people who lose weight also experience increased self-esteem, but they may not experience that weight loss as soon as they experience a spike in energy levels. It may take some time for you to see yourself in your new body and feel better about what you look like.

If you are suffering from low self-confidence, here are some suggestions to help you regain confidence in your weight loss journey. Permit yourself to feel good. Adopt a self-talk habit to proclaim that you have the right to feel good about yourself — even if you are beginning your weight loss journey or haven't reached your weight goal yet. You have the right to feel better about yourself because of the person inside you.

Use words of positivity to promote positive thinking in you. *"I affirm my intelligence." "I affirm my abilities to achieve my aims." "I affirm my choice to be healthy." "I affirm my new energy." "I affirm the energy I have to attain my weight loss ambitions."* Statements such as these give you the power to convert your negative thoughts into positive ones. Get support from others. It is important to accommodate yourself with a community of people who support you on your goals and journey. The people around you affect your feelings. Choose to pass your time with people who increase your self-confidence and self-esteem. Being healthy may be at the top of the list of reasons to lose weight or consider obesity surgery, but when you start your journey to lose that extra weight, lose There are certainly many other weight loss benefits that you will enjoy [47]

Relax Your Relationship with Food

It has been found that people usually don't know how to eat. There are many habits that people adapt. Such adaptations act negatively on their health. Some of them are skipping breakfast, eating in-bulk, nighttime noshing, eating in haste, etc. Suppose we overeat food, or the food gives the body the wrong direction. In that case, we can become overweight, underweight, and put at risk for diseases and conditions like arthritis, diabetes, and heart disease. In short, what we eat is directly related to our health. Consider it in terms of Webster's definition of medicine:

"The science and art dealing with health maintenance and the prevention, alleviation, or cure of disease." [48]

> **Do you know?**
>
> **Protein intake induces the production of dopamine and norepinephrine. Both are brain chemicals and play their role in your mood, motivation, and concentration. The Mediterranean diet, which includes protein-rich edibles, has been significantly crucial for decreasing depression. Consuming a diet that involves whole, unrefined foods with enough protein helps keep blood sugar stable after meals, which has been associated with improvements in mood and anxiety.**

In the short term, a poor diet can contribute to stress, fatigue, and our ability to work and, over time, it can add up to our risk of developing many diseases and conditions.

Other health problems such as:

- ✓ Overweight or obese
- ✓ Tooth decay
- ✓ High Blood Pressure
- ✓ High cholesterol
- ✓ Heart disease and stroke
- ✓ Type 2 diabetes
- ✓ Osteoporosis
- ✓ Some cancers like breast, gallbladder, etc.
- ✓ Depression, anxiety
- ✓ Eating disorders like bulimia and anorexia. [49]

<u>Let's look at some of those eating habits that can cause severe gastric and eating complications that can be fatal.</u>

Mindless Eating

It usually includes eating in large containers or dishes. The size of the dish can make you eat more without focusing. Plate shape and package size, lighting and layout, color, and convenience: are some of the potential persuasive factors that can contribute to the amount of food a person eats. These environmental factors influence eating by increasing consumption norms and reducing consumption monitoring. Moreover, simply raising awareness and providing nutrition education will not be effective in changing mindless eating habits [50]. To counter this habit, you should use small dishes.

Night-time noshing

Timing of intake has been investigated as a novel factor in the aetiology, maintenance, and treatment of obesity. Indeed, eating large amounts of food during the day and night is associated with higher body weight and may even hinder weight loss. The dietary quality of late-night eaters may be a factor in these relationships. Additionally, the nutritional profile of foods eaten at night can negatively affect metabolism and circadian rhythms essential for optimal health [51]. Many nutritionists suggest that eating at night is never a good idea, even if you are losing weight. In this way, the timing of eating is as important as what you are eating.

Skipping Breakfast

Breakfast is the most essential meal of the day and is usually taken after an overnight fast or long rest. Many health surveys and cross-sectional studies have reported the positive effects of breakfast on children's memory recall, functioning, mood, work performance, cognitive function, and women's health, such as irregular menstruation, reduced obesity, and influence on body mass index. However, people worldwide skip breakfast for several reasons: lack of time, home environment, single-family, not being hungry in the morning, or having some misconception like thinking they are fat. Skipping breakfast is bad for your health [52].

Emotional Overeating

Imagine having a misfortune like a breakup or being insulted by the boss or bullied. The negative drive can make you eat delightful dishes like ice cream, chocolate, etc. many types of research have shown that positive and negative feelings can urge you to eat more than your body requires. *"Even at a healthy BMI, emotional overeating can be a problem,"* says Rebekka Schnepper of the University of Salzburg in Austria [53]. Emotional eaters have more robust craving responses and find food more enjoyable when they are in grief than when their emotions are neutral.

Eating in-Haste

Eating quickly is strongly associated with more body weight gaining. Whether snacking or eating a meal, gobbling up food doesn't give your brain time to catch up to your stomach. Your brain doesn't signal that you're full until 15-20 minutes after you start eating. If you swallow your meal in 10 minutes or less, you may eat more than you need. In a study of 3,200 men and women, Japanese researchers found that eating too quickly was strongly associated with being overweight. [54]

If you have gained a lot of weight and want to lose weight, you would probably have these habits. These habits play a crucial role in losing your physique. You got fat, and now, most people don't like you. You might be a victim of body-shaming. So now, it's your decision whether you want to shut those mouths who abuse you just because of your weight or let them abuse you. If you want to silence them, I got a brilliant idea for it. Next, I will talk about the workouts you can do to get your desired physique. I will also show you how you can use those emotions which make you eat to get yourself fit and muscular.

Discover People's Value (Coaching to find out personal values that they must drive to purpose)

Before taking any step further, you need counselling or a coach. You may take the wrong step, either gaining more weight or getting an irregular body shape. Why coaching and counselling are essential? Multiple studies will show you, its importance.

> **Do you know?**
>
> **Research shows that coaching helps you to lose your weight 3 times more than if you act solely or on your own**

Here are some reasons why you need a coach:

- ✓ A weight loss coach will observe your health from an outside perspective, keep you distraction-free, and remind you why you want to lose weight

in the first place. It's easy to get distracted and overwhelmed, putting yourself down and letting negative thoughts cloud your judgment. A good coach will help you to avoid the negative downward spirit.
- ✓ Coaches design your weight loss program to meet your specific needs and find the right balance of nutrition and exercise for your metabolism and lifestyle. There's nothing worse than a diet with the food you don't like or training you don't like. Weight loss coaches ensure that your diet is manageable and your fitness enjoyable.
- ✓ Coaches make you accountable for your workout because it is easy for you to backslide yourself. Coaches identify your goals and help you unleash your potential, and take responsibility for your actions. They are masters of your potential, soundboards for your decisions, and challenges to your blind spots. Ultimately, the coach knows that you want to reach your goals and that holding you accountable is part of the process.
- ✓ Most diets and weight loss plans begin to fail after just a few weeks before completely disappearing. It happens to be our best. There are many reasons, but a weight loss coach will get you off your sofa set and back on track even when you don't want to. You're not the only one experiencing inevitable disappointment. A slimming coach will help you get up and running by being objective and focused.
- ✓ If you skip a workout or backtrack on your diet, a weight loss coach will help get you back. Sometimes life throws a ball at us; More often than not, we tend to use life as an excuse. A weight loss coach will be objective about your problems and make sure that even if you have to skip a workout, you'll catch up and stay more focused going forward [55]

Caching Exercises

Let's move towards some workouts you need to lower your fat from every part of your body. I will recommend some exercises which you can efficiently perform at home. But before that, I would consider it necessary to talk about some misperceptions that people should start with complex exercises. Some also believe that a workout is more important than a diet. Fortunately, none of them is true because nobody would dare to lose weight if they were. Simple basic exercises like jogging and walking can do wonders. Apart from that, a workout without a proper diet is just like a car without an engine-both are useless.

> **Do you know?**
>
> **Walking just 30 minutes every day increase your cardiovascular health, strengthen your bones, reduce extra body fat and boost your muscular health and endurance. Moreover, it also reduces the risk of many diseases like diabetes type 2, blood pressure, and many more.**

<u>Here are some basic exercises which can help you to lose your weight and you can even do them at home:</u>

Burpees

Burpees are the ultimate fat-burning exercise. You work in many muscle groups, including muscles, shoulders, arms, and legs. Plus, you'll sweat and burn some serious calories.

Here is the procedure:

- ✓ Stand with feet shoulder-width apart.
- ✓ Bend your knees and lower your body into a squat, placing your hands between your feet.
- ✓ Bring the leg back to the plank position.
- ✓ Then jump from feet to hands.
- ✓ Raise your arms above your head and jump into the air.
- ✓ Land and immediately drop into a squat on the next rep.
- ✓ Target 10-15 reps.
- ✓ Rest 30 seconds and then repeat three sets [56]

Kettlebell swings

Kettlebell swing has gained popularity as a quick full-body workout. Kettlebells (called girya in Russian) are related with great strength and power over the past decade. They were initially used to measure the weight of various products but were eventually used in strength competitions. These days, they're common in training programs like CrossFit and athletic training programs. This because they are convenient and relatively simple to use, they are also often included in an intense exercise plan for the average person. It mainly targets your posterior chain, i.e., glutes, hamstrings, calves, erector spinae, trapezius (traps), and rhomboids.

Here is how it is done:

- ✓ Stand with your feet shoulder-width apart while holding a kettlebell with both hands (palms facing you) and arms extended straight down.
- ✓ Inhale and push your hips back (hinge hips) and slightly bend your knees to bring the weights between your legs.
- ✓ Make sure to keep your spine straight and focus on your body.
- ✓ Exhale, contract your glutes and push your hips forward to bring your body back to standing. Let your arms swing the weight as far as possible. Shoulder height or parallel to the ground is your goal, although you don't want to use arm strength to lift warm weights. It can take a few turns to find your rhythm and maximize lift.
- ✓ Inhale and lower the warm dumbbells between your legs, pushing your hips back and bending your knees slightly.
- ✓ That is 1 representative. Do 2-3 sets of 10-20 reps each, or continue for any length of time you choose (e.g., as many reps you can do in 5 minutes) [57]

Mountain climbing

Mountain climbing would be a strenuous exercise for most people, but what if mountains were the ground? The same is the concept behind the climbers. Starting from a plank position, you'll alternately bring one knee toward your chest and then out, accelerating until you're "running" on the floor. Although the move sounds simple, climbers exercise almost the entire body and improve your heart rate. You can easily add climbers to your morning workout at home or the gym, in your hotel room when travelling, or even take a few into the break room at work. Fundamental movements are great for beginners, but more experienced users can go a step further with variations.

The procedure for beginners is:

- ✓ Get right into a plank position, ensuring to distribute your weight calmly among your palms and your toes.
- ✓ Check your form—your palms must be approximately shoulder-width apart, flat, abs engaged, and head in alignment.
- ✓ Pull your proper knee into your chest as away as you can.
- ✓ Switch legs, pulling one knee out and bringing the opposite knee in.
- ✓ Keep your hips down and run your knees inside and outside as a way and as rapid as you can. Alternate breathing in and exhaling with every leg change [58]

Renegade rows

Renegade row is a great way to strengthen your back muscles, essential for functional core strength. If you're looking for a way to fit this exercise into a more robust routine, see the Build Your Best Back workout. Renegade row is a powerful movement that strengthens the arms, back, shoulders, and core.

Before we get started, here are some tips for completing the Renegade Row. Tighten the gluteal and abdominal muscles. Tighten your standing legs. Keep your body parallel (do not rotate your hips). You will need dumbbells for this exercise. Columns of dumbbells are complex, so choose weights that add enough resistance to challenge you but not enough to sacrifice foam. Forms are significant for adequate exercise. In today's world, laptops and smartphones tend to be in a bad posture. Our backs are hit hard!

- ✓ Hold the dumbbells in your hands, extend your arms and start with the complete board on your toes. (If you don't have a perfect plank, knee variations are acceptable.) Tighten your abdominal muscles and pull your abdomen inward toward your spine.
- ✓ Keep your weight close to your side and pull up the right dumbbell to the right hip bone. Slowly put it back on the floor and repeat with the dumbbell on the left [59]

Squats

Squats are considered compound exercises. It acts on multiple muscle groups that span multiple joints. The main muscles involved in movement are the quadriceps (the muscle in front of the thigh) and the gluteal muscle (the gluteal muscle). The eccentric part of the movement, the lowering of the squat, also stimulates the hamstrings and hip flexor muscles. Squats also work on the muscles around the knees to help build strength and prevent injuries [60]

Before you do squats, note down these tips:

- ✓ Make your legs slightly wider than your hips, and stand with your toes facing forward.
- ✓ Push your hips back-bend your knees and ankles, and open your knees.
- ✓ Sit on a squat, put your heels and toes on the floor, turn your chest up, and turn your shoulders back.
- ✓ Strive to be parallel in the end. That is, the knee bends at a 90° angle.
- ✓ Push in the heel to straighten your foot and return it to the upright position [61]

You can see above some basic home-based exercises with minimum or no equipment. Remember that a proper diet is also needed to get what type of physique you want. But an important factor is motivation. The coach will motivate you to do the workout, but inner motivation is also needed. I will tell you how to use your emotions to make your workout and diet work. I told you that your food makes you eat it by any means. It plays with your emotions, but I will show you how these emotions can make you lose weight.

The fundamental emotions for the best result

Whenever you try to lose weight at first, you have to make up your mind about it. You get lazy when you are fat. So, the foremost thing is that you emotionally feel to get a muscular body. Emotions play a crucial role in doing any work. For instance, if you do a 9-5 job, why? Because you are motivated that you'll get paid at the end of the month. You need to get motivated to turn your hanging belly into a muscular one.

How do emotions work?

Every day, our emotions face us with an enduring mystery. On the one hand, emotions that seem out of our control come to us. We may be angry, embarrassed, hysterically grabbed by something we find interesting, or crying with joy [62]. What comes to your mind first when you think about losing weight? If you're like most people, the answer would be diet and exercise. Apart from these crucial factors, other factors can lead to weight loss planning or breaking.

When people embark on a weight loss journey, the emotional aspect of weight loss is often lost. Emotions determine our lives in different ways. We act unknowingly in areas that affect weight, such as eating emotionally, relieving pain, or reducing food intake to reach weight goals. Emotional diets are perceived as compulsive behaviour and are evidence that our emotional state can affect our diet. How we eat affects our weight loss and weight gain. It is widespread to have a training partner for training. It's not uncommon for people to start a diet with friends for support.

We know that this support can often contribute to the success of exercise and weight loss programs. These forms of support can support the emotional part of a weight loss journey. Having someone to share the experience can energize us when we haven't reached our commitment to lose weight. Plans with a sound support system will also benefit from goal setting. Smart goals are a great way to help us along the way to successful and sustainable weight loss. Find the best you can support, set your goals and continue your journey to improve your health [63].

When losing weight, you can face many psychological blocks. These hurdles are a leading factor behind your disheartening. When it comes to eating habits, it's challenging to change your habits. Our bodies are designed for food, and we need it to survive. Eating will make you feel better. Most of us have good intentions regarding proper diet and more frequent exercise. And most of us know what to eat and what to avoid.

However, it often stops progressing when tired, stressed, bored, or frustrated, even with the best intentions. These feelings come out a lot. We are all habitual creatures. We find comfort in our daily lives. Therefore, if your routine contains patterns of diet and activity that lead to unhealthy weight, it is common to look for those simple habits when the situation becomes severe. These habits relieve symptoms, at least in the short term. To make matters worse, you may have powerful rationalization skills that help you perpetuate unhealthy habits. After all, why do you give up the practice of providing relief and comfort? [64]

The following could be some tips to overcome psychological barriers:

1. **Keep a Daily Journal.** It is not always possible to avoid stress. However, you can identify the triggers of stress and do your best to avoid certain situations and people that undermine your success. Keeping a diary may be helpful. Studies show that keeping a diary can double the results of weight loss. There are many ways to use the diary. For example, just record your dietary intake in your diary. However, you can also use it to write down your thoughts and try to identify the trigger for stress. Use the journal to track situations and foods that you feel are triggering you. Would you like to overeat or eat unhealthy food when you are in a particular environment or around certain people? Can you identify specific situations that are out of control and require comfort? Keeping a diary can help you identify these situations to limit or avoid your exposure ultimately.

2. **Make Small Changes.** If all-or-nothing thinking prevents you from sticking to your food plan, consider taking small steps and setting short goals. First, find out one specific healthy change that is reasonable and attainable. Perhaps you can choose to walk for 20 minutes after dinner every day. Set a goal and path to follow on that target for a week. If you keep a diary, write down notes each day about how you have successfully kept that goal in front of your mind. And respect yourself. Remember that taking small steps is way better than taking bigger steps or not taking a step at all. You can also take small steps to avoid making many changes at once. If you do a lot at once, you tend to lose motivation. Instead, if you can make small changes well, you can enjoy a rewarding sense of accomplishment. Remind yourself that being perfect is not the goal, but an attempt to nudge yourself in the right direction is progress you should be proud of in the end.

3. **Listen to your inner self**. Do you bother yourself to pay attention to the signals you send yourself throughout the day? These negative thoughts can be a barrier to successful weight loss. People prone to negative body image may repeat negative messages about their bodies throughout the day. Sentences like "I'm too fat" or "I'm so unbalanced" said aloud or in your head can interfere with your ability to take healthy action when given the opportunity. Self-talk is another way all-or-nothing thinking can work. For example, you may blame yourself for meeting unreasonably high standards or aims that you set for yourself. Take a week or more to listen to your inner conversation. Identify one or two messages that might encourage a negative self-image and write them down. You can then challenge them or replace these messages with a powerful spell. Phrases like *"my body is strong," "I've had enough,"* or *"I've come a long way"* are common mantras used to build confidence.
4. **Learn Relaxation Techniques**. If you can't avoid stressful people or places, relaxation techniques can be a healthy alternative to managing emotions during stress. Scientists have found that a specific type of relaxation technique, called guided imagery, can help with weight loss. You can work with a therapist to learn how imagery can help you lose weight. Instructions, but images can be learned under your own guidance. It takes time to master, but guided imagery can be the most effective weight loss technique if emotions force you to eat during times of stress.
5. **Prioritize Sleep**. Researchers have repeatedly found a link between sleep habits, stress, depression, and an unhealthy diet. One of the most straightforward and relaxing steps you can take to break down psychological barriers is to improve your sleep habits. Make your bedroom a sleeping paradise. Remove electronic devices (TVs, computers, cell phone chargers) and do whatever you can to reduce noise. Get a blackout curtain or buy a cheap sleep mask and experience total darkness at night. Some people lower the thermostat to promote a good night's sleep. Go to bed simultaneously every night and wake up simultaneously every morning.

After all the discussion, you can come to a single point: a fitness triangle contains emotions on top while the workout and diet occupy the lower part. Let me make something clear. When you go to lose weight, you will hit the gym. You will go one day, return, and see no change. You will go again, return without noticing any change, and the cycle will go on. But remember, those good things take time to happen. Empires do not form in a single day. Once you have decided to get your ideal body physique, whether muscular (for men) or slim (for women), you have to stick to it until you get what you want. And one last thing, remember the line from the movie *"Rocky," "there is no tomorrow."* So, if you have decided to work on your health, start doing it now.

CHAPTER #5 - DIET AND SPORTS

We have already discussed some basic workouts, which are easier and can be performed at home. But as it is said before, exercises are good for nothing if they are not accompanied by a perfect diet plan. I will also talk about some outdoor games which can be really helpful for you. A regular physical activity is important for your health, especially if you are trying to lose weight or maintain a healthy weight. When you lose weight, more physical activity increases the number of calories your body uses for energy, or *"burns"*. Burning calories through physical activity combined with reducing the number of calories you eat create a "calorie deficiency" that leads to weight loss. Most weight loss is caused by a decrease in calorie intake.

However, there is evidence that the only way to maintain the weight loss is to do regular physical activity. Most importantly, physical activity reduces the risk of cardiovascular disease and diabetes beyond the risks associated only with weight loss. Physical activity also helps maintain weight. Lowers high blood pressure. Reduces the risk of type 2 diabetes, heart attack, stroke, and various types of cancer. It reduces the pain of arthritis and the associated disorders. Reduces the risk of osteoporosis and falls. It reduces the symptoms of depression and anxiety [65].

While each weight-reduction plan and workout are crucial for weight reduction, it's normally simpler to control your calorie consumption through editing your weight-reduction plan than its miles to burn substantially greater energy thru the workout. This can be why the 80/20 rule has to turn out to be popular because it states that weight reduction is the end result of an 80% weight-reduction plan and a 20% workout. For example, if you are aiming for an everyday calorie deficit of 500 energy, you can eat four hundred less energy (80%) by consuming decreased calorie dishes, smaller element sizes, and fewer snacks.

Then, you best want to burn one hundred energy (20%) from the workout. For many people, that is simpler than seeking to burn 500 energy every day from the workout. Burning this many calories each day calls for a large quantity of movement — plus, it's time-consuming, taxing to the body, and infrequently sustainable. To illustrate, someone who weighs 154 pounds (70 kg) might want to cycle on a workout motorcycle for 1 hour at slight depth to burn 525 energies. Meanwhile, they may reduce 520 energies by skipping out on a venti Green Tea Frappuccino from Starbucks. A clean manner to control calorie consumption and sell weight reduction without counting energy is to pay attention to consuming whole, minimally processed meals which can be excessive in fiber, protein, and healthful fats [66]

Are You a Smoker? Loss Weight Better

Everyone knows that smoking can cause many chronic diseases. And if it accompanies obesity, it can cause disasters that cannot be imagined. According to a study, the life expectancy of obese smokers is 13 years less than that of normal-weight smokers. Another study indicates that 1/3rd to ½ of obese smokers die between 40 to 70 years of age.

You would probably be surprised to know that smokers usually are thinner than nonsmokers. Smoking's impact on body weight ought to cause weight reduction with the aid of growing the metabolic rate, lowering metabolic efficiency, or lowering caloric absorption (discount in appetite), all of which might be related to tobacco use. The metabolic impact of smoking ought to explain the decreased frame weight determined in people who smoke.

Smoking just one cigarette has been proven to set off a 3% upward thrust in EE inside 30 min. Smoking four cigarettes which contain 0.8 mg nicotine each elevated resting EE with the aid of using 3.3 % for three hours. In everyday people who smoke whose metabolism becomes assessed in a metabolic ward, smoking 24 cigarettes in 1 day elevates the overall EE from 2230 to 2445 kcal/d, and stimulation of the sympathetic nervous system activity can be involved. The impact of smoking on EE becomes weaker amongst overweight subjects, and it additionally relies on the degree of body activities and fitness [67]

These studies suggest that smoking is undoubtedly associated with body weight and that heavy people who smoke are much more likely to be obese or overweight than mild people who smoke. These observations are hardly ever acknowledged, and they propose that elements related to smoking counter or even overtake the metabolic impact of smoking.

The query regarding the reason why heavy people who smoke generally tend to have extra body weight than mild people who smoke or are nonsmokers stays unanswered. One rationalization might be that heavy people who smoke are much more likely to undertake behaviors favoring weight gain (e.g., low bodily pastime, dangerous diet, and excessive alcohol intake) than are mild people who smoke or nonsmokers. Smokers consume much less fruit and vegetables, undertake dangerous nutrient intake styles, drink more alcohol, and interact in much less bodily pastime than nonsmokers. We have diagnosed a robust clustering of chance behaviors (i.e., common bodily pastime, low intakes of fruit and vegetables, and excessive alcohol intake) that correlated with the extent of cigarette consumption. Therefore, you must work on losing weight.

Let's discuss some diets which can help you with that.

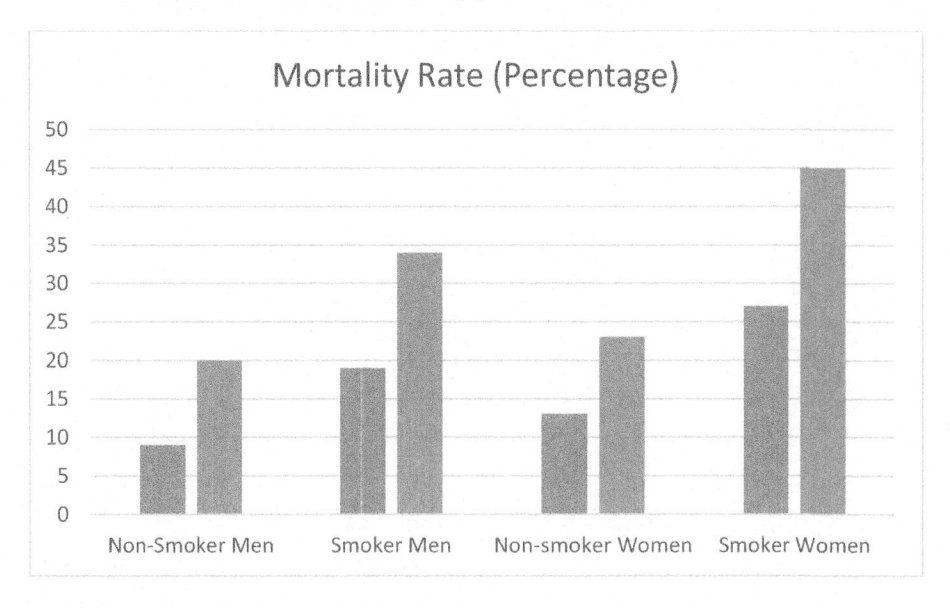

Mortality Rate (Percentage)

Category	Percentage
Non-Smoker Men	9
Non-Smoker Men	20
Smoker Men	19
Smoker Men	34
Non-smoker Women	13
Non-smoker Women	23
Smoker Women	27
Smoker Women	45

Diets that work

Dieting isn't just for weight loss. While changing your diet can be one of the best ways to lose weight, it can also be a gateway to improving your habits, focusing on your health, and having a healthy lifestyle. More active life.

However, the many diet plans available can make it difficult to get started. Different diets are more appropriate, long-lasting, and effective for different people. Some diets are intended to curb your appetite to reduce your food intake.

On the contrary, others suggest limiting your calories and carbohydrates or fats. Some focus more on certain eating habits and lifestyle changes rather than restricting certain foods. In addiction, many offers health benefits beyond just weight loss [68]

Here are some of the best diets to help improve your overall health. We will also discuss their benefits and disadvantages so that you can understand which plan suits you. *Read them carefully and keep in mind your body type and your actual psychological problem.*

1. The Mediterranean Diet

The Mediterranean diet has long been recognized as the gold standard for nutrition, disease prevention, health and longevity. It is based on its nutritional benefits and sustainability. The Mediterranean diet is based on the food traditionally eaten by people from countries such as Italy and Greece. It's abundant in:

- ✓ Vegetables
- ✓ Fruits
- ✓ Full-grain
- ✓ Fish
- ✓ Nuts
- ✓ Lens
- ✓ Olive oil

Foods such as chicken, eggs and dairy products must be consumed in moderation, and lean meat is limited. In addition, the Mediterranean diet restricts:

- ✓ Refined grains
- ✓ Trans-fat
- ✓ Processed meat

- ✓ Added sugar
- ✓ Other highly processed foods

This diet is associated with a reduced risk of some chronic illnesses and an increase in life expectancy by focusing on minimally processed foods and plants. Studies also show that a Mediterranean diet protects against certain types of cancer. Although the diet is designed to reduce the risk of heart disease, many studies have shown that plant-based diet patterns high in unsaturated fats can also contribute to weight loss. A systematic review of five studies found that a Mediterranean diet resulted in greater weight loss in one year compared to a low-fat diet. Compared to a low-carb diet, it resulted in similar weight loss. A 12-month study of more than 500 adults found that higher adherence to a Mediterranean diet was twice as likely to maintain weight loss.

Additionally, the Mediterranean diet promotes the intake of antioxidant-rich foods that may help combat inflammation and oxidative stress by neutralizing free radicals. Recent studies have also found that a Mediterranean diet is associated with a reduced risk of cognitive decline and mental disorders such as depression. Reducing meat intake is associated with a more sustainable diet for the planet.

The Mediterranean diet does not place much emphasis on dairy products, so it is important to have enough calcium and vitamin D in your diet [69]

2. The DASH Diet

DASH stands for Dietary Approaches to Stop Hypertension. The Dash Diet is a healthy diet used to treat or prevent high blood pressure (Hypertension). The Dash Diet contains foods rich in potassium, calcium and magnesium. These nutrients help control blood pressure. Diets limit foods high in sodium, saturated fats, and added sugars. According to studies, the DASH diet can lower blood pressure in just two weeks. Diet can also lower low-density lipoprotein (LDL, or "bad") cholesterol levels in the blood. High blood pressure and high LDL cholesterol are two major risk factors for heart disease and stroke.

This shows the recommended serving of each food group on the DASH diet with 2,000 calories per day.

- ✓ **Grain**: 6-8 servings per day. One serving is a loaf of bread, an ounce of dried granola or cooked granola, rice, and ½ cup of pasta.
- ✓ **Vegetables**: 4-5 servings a day. Serving is 1 cup of raw green leafy vegetables, ½ cup of chopped raw or cooked vegetables, or 1/2 cup of vegetable juice.
- ✓ **Fruits**: 4-5 servings per day. Serving is one medium fruit, 1/2 cup fresh, frozen, or canned fruit, or 1/2 cup fruit juice.
- ✓ **Non-fat or low-fat dairy products**: 2-3 servings daily. Serving is 1 cup of milk, yoghurt, or 1 1/2 ounces of cheese.
- ✓ **Lean meat, chicken, fish**: 6 servings less than 1 ounce daily. Serving is an ounce of cooked meat, chicken, fish, or an egg.
- ✓ **Nuts, seeds, legumes**: 4-5 servings a week. Servings are 1/3 cup nuts, 2 cups peanut butter, 2 cups seeds, or 1/2 cup of cooked legumes (dried or peas).
- ✓ **Oils and fats**: 2-3 servings a day. Serving is 1 teaspoon of soft margarine, 1 teaspoon of vegetable oil, 1 tablespoon of mayonnaise, or 2 tablespoons of salad dressing.
- ✓ **Added sugar and sweets**: 5 meals or less per week. Serving is 1 tablespoon of sugar, jelly or jam, 1/2 cup of sorbet, or 1 cup of soda. [70]

The Dash diet can help people with hypertension to lose weight and lower their blood pressure. Still, there is plenty of evidence about salt intake and blood pressure. Too little salt increases insulin resistance, and a low-salt diet is not the right choice for everyone. Low sodium diets, such as the DASH diet, are suitable for people with high blood pressure or other health conditions benefiting from or need sodium restriction.

3. Flexitarian Diet

If you're looking for a healthy diet that doesn't involve calorie counting, has very strict rules, and can sometimes enjoy meat. You don't have to look for anything more than a flexitarian diet. By its simplest definition, a flexitarian diet combines the words "flexible" and "vegetarian." It's a cross between vegans and vegetarians, and sometimes you have the option to enjoy animal foods. A flexitarian diet is essentially a flexible alternative to being a vegetarian. So, you're still focusing on fruits, vegetables, whole grains, legumes, and nuts, but you still enjoy meat from time to time. If vegetarianism wasn't attractive to you because you love good burgers, a flexitarian diet might be just for you. (Still, it's worth noting that this diet focuses on reducing your overall meat consumption.)

The flexitarian diet is intended to be inclusive. Still, we want to limit animal protein (including seafood) and processed foods and beverages.

Here's what you can add to your cart:

- ✓ Fruit.
- ✓ Vegetable.
- ✓ Plant-based proteins (black, kidney, navy beans, edamame, chickpeas, lentils, tofu).
- ✓ Whole grains (brown rice, oats, barley, quinoa).
- ✓ Vegetable milk (although cow milk is reasonably OK).
- ✓ Eggs.
- ✓ Dairy products (cheese, yoghurt, or milk alternatives).
- ✓ Nuts, nut butter, seeds, healthy fats. Oils, herbs, spices.

What food to limit:

Meat and chicken (lean beef, chicken breast, and turkey breast).

Fish (salmon, tilapia, cod, and shrimp).

Addition of sugar or refined carbohydrates. [71]

4. Mediterranean-DASH Intervention for Neurodegenerative Delay Diet

Mediterranean-DASH Intervention for Neurodegenerative Delay Diet or MIND diet aims to reduce dementia and the decline in brain health that often occurs as people age. It combines aspects of two very popular diets, the Mediterranean diet and the DASH (Dietary Approaches to Preventing Hypertension) diet. Many experts consider the Mediterranean and DASH diets to be among the healthiest. Research has shown that they can lower blood pressure and reduce the risk of heart disease, diabetes, and other diseases. But researchers wanted to create a special diet to help improve brain function and prevent dementia. To do this, they combined Mediterranean foods and the DASH diet, which has been shown to benefit brain health. For example, the Mediterranean diet and DASH recommend eating lots of fruit. Fruit consumption was not correlated with improved brain function, but berry consumption did. The MIND diet, therefore, encourages its followers to eat berries but does not emphasize fruit consumption in general.

Following are foods you can eat while having a MIND diet:

- ✓ **Green leafy vegetables**: Aim for six or more servings per week. This includes kale, spinach, cooked greens, and salads.
- ✓ **All other vegetables**: Try to eat vegetables other than green leafy vegetables at least once a day. It is best to choose non-starchy vegetables as they are high in nutrients and low in calories.
- ✓ **Berries**: Eat berries at least twice a week. Although the published research only included strawberries, you should also eat other berries like blueberries, blackberries, and blackberries for their antioxidant benefits
- ✓ **Nuts**: Aim to eat five or more servings of nuts per week. The creators of the MIND diet don't specify which nuts to eat, but it's probably best to vary the nuts you eat to get more nutrients.
- ✓ **Olive oil**: Use olive oil as the main cooking oil. Check out this article for more information on the safety of cooking with olive oil.
- ✓ **Whole grains**: Aim for at least three servings per day. Choose whole grains like rolled oats, quinoa, brown rice, whole-wheat pasta, and 100% whole-wheat bread.
- ✓ **Fish**: Eat fish at least once a week. It is better to choose fatty fish such as salmon, sardines, trout, tuna and mackerel as they are high in omega3 fatty acids.
- ✓ **Beans**: Include beans in at least four meals a week. This includes all beans, lentils and soybeans.
- ✓ **Poultry**: Try to eat chicken or turkey at least twice a week. Note that fried chicken is not recommended on the MIND diet.
- ✓ **Wine**: Do not drink more than one drink per day. Both red and white wine are beneficial for the brain. However, much research has focused on the red wine compound resveratrol, which may help protect against Alzheimer's disease [72]

5. Weight Watchers

Weight Watchers is one of the world's most popular weight loss programs. While it doesn't restrict any food groups, people following the WW diet should eat within their daily score to help them reach their ideal weight. WW is a points-based system that assigns a value to foods and beverages based on their calorie, fat, and fiber content. When trying to reach your desired weight, you must stay within your daily allowance. Many studies show that the WW program can help you lose weight.

For example, a review of 45 studies found that people who followed the WW diet lost 2.6% more weight than those who received standard advice. In addition, people following the WW program are more successful at maintaining weight loss after several years than those following other diets. WW allows flexibility, making tracking easier. This allows people with dietary restrictions, such as food allergies, to join the program.

While it does allow for flexibility, WW can be expensive depending on the subscription plan and how long you plan to follow it. Studies show that significant weight loss and clinical benefits can take up to 52 weeks. Also, its versatility can be a drawback if dieters choose unhealthy foods. [73]

6. Irregular Fasting

Intermittent fasting means that you don't eat for a certain amount of time each day or week.

Some common approaches to intermittent fasting include:

- ✓ Eat a normal diet one day and fast completely or a small meal (less than 500 calories) the next day.
- ✓ Fasting 5: 2. Eat a normal diet five days a week and fast two days a week.
- ✓ Daily fasting has a time limit. Eat normally, but only for 8 hours a day. For example, skip breakfast but eat lunch around noon and dinner around 8pm.

Some studies show that alternate-day fasting is as effective as a typical low-calorie diet for weight loss. This seems reasonable because reducing your calorie intake will help you lose weight.

Some studies suggest intermittent fasting may be more beneficial than other diets in reducing inflammation and improving inflammation-related conditions.

Example:

- ✓ Alzheimer's disease
- ✓ Arthritis
- ✓ Asthma
- ✓ Multiple sclerosis stroke

It is important to note that intermittent fasting can cause unpleasant side effects but usually disappears within a month.

The possible side effects are:

- ✓ Hunger
- ✓ Malaise
- ✓ Insomnia
- ✓ Nausea
- ✓ Headache [74]

> **Do you know?**
> **In general, intermittent fasting is safe for most healthy adults. However, people who are sensitive to low blood sugar levels should consult a doctor before starting an intermittent fast. These groups include people:**

- Suffering from diabetes
- Lightweight People with eating disorders
- Pregnant women
- Women who are breastfeeding

7. The Volumetric Diet

The Volumetrics diet claims to help you feel full while eating fewer calories. Based on the book of Nutritionists, Dr. Barbara Rolls contains detailed guidelines, recipes, and information on calculating the calorie density of your favorite foods. The diet recommends eating nutritious foods low in calories and water, such as fruits, vegetables and soups. On the other hand, limit high-calorie foods such as cookies, candies, nuts, seeds and oils. Dr. Rolls claims that these restrictions help you feel full longer, reduce calorie intake, and promote weight loss. Unlike other diets, the Volumetrics diet is designed to promote a healthy diet and should be seen as a long-term lifestyle change rather than a short-term solution. The Volumetrics diet is designed to help you feel full while eating fewer calories.

Volumetrics Diet classifies foods into four categories based on calorie density.

- ✓ **Category 1** (Very low-calorie density): Calorie density less than 0.6. It includes Starch-free fruits and vegetables, non-fat milk, broth-based soup
- ✓ **Category 2** (low calorie density): 0.6-1.5 calorie density. It involves Starch fruits and vegetables, grains, breakfast cereals, lean meats, low-calorie foods such as legumes, low-fat mixed foods such as chili
- ✓ **Category 3** (intermediate calorie density): 1.6-3.9 calorie density. It contains medium-calorie foods such as meat, cheese, pizza, bread and ice cream
- ✓ **Category 4** (high-calorie density): 4.0-9.0 calorie density. It includes Crackers, chips, chocolate, nuts, butter, and oil [75]

While the Volumetrics diet is effective for health benefits and weight loss, it requires a good understanding of Volumetrics, including learning about the caloric content of food serving size and nutrient levels.

Sport Ways for Weight Loss

Everyone in this world has a dream of getting an athletic body. It's not that easy. It requires hard work and persistence. Weight is a recent issue that has been attracting attention due to major illness-causing problems such as obesity, heart disease, and fatigue. Indulging in these fat-burning sports will also sharpen your mind and memory. Following are some sports which can help you to lose weight.

Swimming

The biggest health benefit of swimming is that it doesn't affect your joints at all, and it's a great tonic. Swimmers use every muscle to propel themselves through the water, including the neck, face, and toes. It builds muscle strength and courage while improving posture and flexibility. Swimming also provides an effective aerobic exercise. Swimming provides the cardiovascular benefits of aerobic exercise without putting much strain on your joints. Age, injury, or obesity-related conditions may cause you to choose a sport that puts no stress on your body [76]

> **Do you know?**
>
> **Swimming for 1 hour burns almost 500 to 800 calories**

Running

Running is an extremely effective fat-burning exercise. In fact, when it comes to weight loss, it's hard to beat. It is estimated that running for 1 hour burns 900 to 1500 calories. According to data from the American Council on Exercise, a 180-pound runner burns 170 calories running at a steady pace for 10 minutes. Run for 30 minutes, and that runner will burn over 500 calories. But just running long won't help you lose belly fat. You also need to change your diet and lifestyle to address these issues. If you want to see the results, you have to be trained and do it difficultly. To get rid of stubborn tummy fat, moderate-intensity activity 4-5 times a week for up to 30-60 minutes. It sounds like a daunting task, and finding time can be difficult when you have a busy schedule. [77]

Racquetball

Those interested in racquetball need a good hand, eye coordination, and cardiovascular durability to support the game. The game is very addictive and entertaining, as evidenced by the fact that the focus on training is forgotten during the overall experience of this fast-paced game. An hourly racquetball can burn up to 600,800 calories. Players can run more than 2 miles in a single game. It's called aerobic exercise because it keeps your heart rate at about 70-80% of your maximum capacity. The harder a person plays, the harder their heart works, and the more calories they burn. Regular racquetball will help you maintain a healthy weight by steadily reducing your body fat percentage. This is a great core workout, and if you play it regularly, you'll get immediate results for anyone who wants to lose extra weight [78]

Soccer

Soccer is the best sport to lose weight because it makes your muscles and heart work differently. Soccer builds muscle mass and burns fat by mobilizing muscle fibers in both slow and fast spasms. As an aerobic exercise, playing soccer consumes more calories than regular workouts because it forces you to alternate between aerobic and anaerobic energy pathways. Unlike some aerobic exercises, soccer does not promote muscle destruction but builds and maintains muscle mass and increases metabolism.

A game of soccer burns about 260 calories in just 30 minutes for a 155 pounds person. To lose weight, you need to burn more calories. Specifically, you need to burn 3,500 calories to lose 1 pound of fat. So, if you play soccer three times a week for an hour, you burn an additional 1,500 calories each week, and you can lose 2 pounds a month on soccer alone. Aerobic and anaerobic exercises are used in football games because you always have to exercise at different intensity levels. By constantly switching between these energy systems, you burn more calories.

According to the University of Copenhagen, playing soccer regularly has been shown to reduce body fat. In soccer games, soccer works with fast muscle fibers because it uses explosive power for sprinting, jumping, turning, and other explosive movements. Fast-twitch fiber requires stored glucose for energy, so it releases fat-burning hormones that continue to burn fat during and after exercise. This allows you to burn more fat than training slow-twitch fiber with regular aerobic exercise.

Playing soccer activates both fast spasm fibers during explosive movements and slow, spasmodic fibers during aerobic exercise. Working more muscle fibers causes more muscles. Stimulates growth. Soccer uses all major muscle groups to challenge the gluteal muscles, hamstrings, quadriceps, calves, etc., especially the lower body. The more muscle you have, the higher your metabolism. Therefore, if you are building your major muscle groups efficiently, you will also burn fatter from the field. [79]

Basketball

Basketball may not be the most efficient way to lose weight, but it is very effective. Those who dislike rigorous and demanding activities such as running may find basketball useful because it combines fun and friendly competition with the ability to burn calories. Adjusting your diet and spending enough time and effort can help basketball lose fat.

When trying to lose weight, one of the motivations for exercising may be to burn more calories than you burn. According to Michigan State University, this is called a calorie deficit. Diet is also important in weight loss because it can be difficult to create a calorie deficit if you consume too many calories. The calories' quality of the calories matters too. You should eat a healthy diet filled with whole foods rich in fiber to nourish your body and suppress hunger. Calories Burned Playing Basketball according to Harvard Medical School, a 155-pound person can burn around 288 calories in 30 minutes of playing basketball. However, a person with a higher body weight may expend more energy: A 185-pound individual can burn about 336 calories in 30 minutes of basketball.

Comparing calorie consumption, most sports, including basketball, starts and stop. They may require considerable effort to play, but they may not burn as many calories as continuous exercises such as strenuous running or cycling. For example, Harvard Medical School says 155-pound people running at 7.5 miles per hour can burn 450 calories in 30 minutes. However, 155-pound people cycling at 16-19 miles per hour can burn about 432 calories in 30 minutes. [80]

Boxing

Boxing has existed for centuries as a form of martial arts and solo sportsI. Some people do it as part of their training program while doing it as self-defense. People are usually attracted to boxing because it's fun and fun. In addition, it guarantees a dramatic improvement in well-being and overall health. Boxing is incredible for anyone who wants to lose weight.

Boxing is a high-impact aerobic exercise that provides significant calories burning. Cardio boxing burns more calories than other types of cardiovascular exercises. A typical boxing session can burn up to 1000 calories. Compared to other exercises, such as walking (243 calories), jogging (398 calories) and running (544 calories), the calorie consumption of a boxing session overpowers all of them. If you want to lose weight faster and reach your weight loss goals faster, boxing exercises are for you.

Boxing is a serious calorie burner, but it's also very effective at burning fat. The high intensity of boxing training means that it is very good at burning visceral fat, or fat that is commonly found around the waist. Not all fats are made the same. Tummy fat is associated with toxins that change how the body works and increase the risk of various illnesses. Tummy fat is associated with an increased risk of diabetes, heart disease, and certain types of cancer, such as esophageal, colon, and pancreatic cancer. Boxing is a great way to reduce visceral fat and the associated medical risks around the waist.

It's easy to get bored with your workout when there's not much variety in your work. Let's face it, jumping on the treadmill day in and day out or walking briskly on the same path can quickly get boring. Plus, such exercises don't give you the full-body workout you need for optimal bodybuilding and weight loss. Boxing workouts work your entire body, engaging all your muscle groups to increase the intensity of your workout and help you lose weight faster. With continuous speed boxing, ball punching, jumping rope and resistance training built into most boxing workouts, you won't need to add much to your daily exercise routine in order to achieve the desired results. [81]

Cycling

Cycling is frequently touted as a terrific low-effect alternative for cardio exercising. It lets you get your coronary heart rate up with much less put on and tear for your knees, ankles, and different joints compared to jogging or running. It's additionally a terrific manner that will help you shed more pounds. That's because you could burn an outstanding variety of energy even as you're pedaling, mainly in case you cycle past a leisurely pace.

Indoors

Do you opt to exercise indoors? Here are more than one approaches to motorcycle inside:

- ✓ Ride a desk-bound cycle for your personal. Whether you own a desk-bound motorcycle or operate one at a fitness center, you could get an exceptional exercise tailor-made for your needs. Many programmable alternatives allow you to customize your exercise to the speed, depth, and length you need.
- ✓ Spin classes. If you want a person to inspire you to hold on to using via your exercise, this is probably a terrific choice. Research Trusted Source additionally shows that spinning is simply as powerful for enhancing your bodily health and converting your body as compared with normal bicycle use.
- ✓ Hand cycle. Suppose you're now no longer capable of using a normal desk-bound bicycle. In that case, a hand cycle is probably needed for a few calorie-burning cardio exercising. This system is powered using your hands as opposed to your legs.

You'll ensure to get admission to a desk-bound motorcycle or hand cycle in case you move this route. If you do not own your personal equipment, you need to inspect becoming a fitness or community center member.

Outdoors

If you opt to take your bicycle out into the exceptional outdoors, you've got numerous alternatives, including street cycling, path cycling, or mountain cycling. You should even ditch your bike and attempt cycling to paintings or using your motorcycle to run errands. But it can't be a one-time thing. You want to make cycling a normal part of your exercise habitual in case you need to apply this sort of exercise to lose weight. You can track your mileage or depth with various apps too. Using a health monitoring app can also assist you in living stimulated to attain precise goals. The one drawback to outdoor cycling is that you want to observe greater protection precautions to keep living securely. Wet, icy, or choppy street situations, warm or humid weather, and unpredictable visitor situations could make outside cycling much less secure than biking indoors. [82]

Personalize Your Best Food Plan

There is no single rule that fits all obese persons. Still, to lose weight at a safe and sustainable rate of 0.5-1 kg per week, most people reduce their energy intake by 600 calories per day is recommended. For most men, this means consuming less than 1,900 calories per day, and for most women, consuming less than 1,400 calories per day. The best way to do this is to replace unhealthy, high-energy foods such as fast foods, processed foods, and sweet drinks (including alcohol) with healthier alternatives.

A healthy diet should consist of:

- ✓ Lots of fruits and vegetables
- ✓ Lots of potatoes, bread, rice, pasta and other starchy foods (ideally, choose whole grains)
- ✓ Some milk and dairy products
- ✓ Some non-dairy protein sources such as meat, fish, eggs, beans, and other dairy products
- ✓ Only small amounts of high-fat and high-carbohydrate foods and beverages

Whenever you begin to follow your diet plan, make sure you follow these tips:

- ✓ Try to eat more soluble fiber like berries, legumes etc.
- ✓ Avoid such food which contains trans-fat, which can be found in margarine, spreads, and other packed and processed foods
- ✓ Avoid drinking alcohol. If you are an addict, then reduce your consumption
- ✓ Try to make your diet enriched with pretentious food
- ✓ Try to remain calm and relax yourself
- ✓ Lower your sugar consumption
- ✓ Do cardio exercises like cycling, running, swimming etc.
- ✓ Avoid carbs. More specifically, refined carbs
- ✓ Get plenty of sleep (almost 8 hours a day)
- ✓ Perform fasting once a week
- ✓ Add green tea to your diet

You must be aware of your diets, sports and workouts suitable for you. It is up to you to recognize yourself and plan your diet according to it. You have gone through various dietary programs. But, remember that there is no strict obligation on you to strictly follow any single of them. You can edit your plan, but coach consultation is obligatory. Moreover, try to keep yourself hydrated and get enough sleep as a sound body has a sound mind.

CHAPTER #6 – STRATEGIES

We have discussed several strategies useful to lose weight like overcoming your psychological barrier, maintaining your diet plan, workouts, and sports which can be effective in losing weight. But now, I will tell you about something more that can help you become self-motivated. You might be wondering what is left behind after the traditional ways. You might be thinking that you overpowered my mind, you are strictly following the prescribed diet, etc., and so what is this new thing. It's Neuro-Linguistic Programming, aka NLP. Neuro-linguistic programming (NLP) examines the gears in a machine, the human mind. It helps to understand what promotes human behavior. It focuses on how our thoughts, behaviors, emotions, and many other individual characteristics are combined to influence our actions [83]

I will also show you how visualization can be an effective tool to counter your overweight. Because when you see different body types like shredded or athletic, you desire to gain those amazing forms. If you are confused about what visualization means, looking up the definition in a dictionary can leave you with many other questions. The Merriam-Webster Dictionary defines visualization as *"the formation of mental or action visual images or the process of interpreting visual terms or bringing them into visible form."* If you're like most people, this definition probably does not reveal much about you. A simplified version of the definition of visualization is: imagine in your head what you want out of your life. Visualization is often associated with meditation and mindfulness. What the process should be like, go to a quiet place, close your eyes and calm your body and start thinking about what you want to experience in life. You want to get as much detail as possible [84].

NLP Restructuring Exercise

Neurolinguistic programming studies how our thoughts affect our behavior. It examines how our brain interprets the signals it receives and how those interpretations affect our actions. It does this through language - the linguistic part of Neurolinguistic programming. By examining how our brains process information, NLP techniques help us see our thoughts, feelings, and emotions as things, we can control rather than things that happen to us. [85]

Let's understand how NLP works by using a simple example. Imagine your brain as a computer with lots of wires. These wires contain all the data collected from your life experience, resulting in your *"mind map."* You look different from the next person. Filters in your world (mind) have been conditioned by your parents, culture, and education in many other personal experiences. Sometimes the way you see the world is in your interest. For example, when you see the positive and good things in everything that happens or the opportunities that happen in all situations. However, these "wires" in the brain may be programmed to provoke anxiety (or worse, phobia) reactions to the situation, destroy self-confidence, or lead to bad habits. [86]

NLP uses perceptual, behavioral, and communication techniques to make it easy for people to change their thoughts and behaviors. NLP relies on language processing but should not be confused with natural language processing that uses the same acronym. The NLP was developed by Richard Bandler and John Grinder, who believed it was possible to successfully identify people's patterns of thought and behavior and teach them to others. Despite the lack of empirical evidence, Bundler and Grinder have published two books, *"Magic Structures I and II,"* and NLP has taken off. Its popularity was partly due to its versatility in dealing with people's many problems. [87]

Theory of NLP

NLP with techniques strongly influenced by hypnosis, psychotherapy, and psychology. Ericksonian Hypnosis and Classical Conditioning are two prominent examples. They "modelled" the things that worked the fastest and seemed to have the best patient results and combined them to create what is now known as Neuro-Linguistic Programming. The theoretical basis of NLP techniques has been supported by research in psychology. A major example is a phenomenon known as "submodules" in NLP. Not all techniques have been thoroughly studied. Frequently asked the question: "Is NLP real?" While it may sound a little over the top, the claims about NLP have been confirmed and successfully applied in the field of psychotherapy [88]

How NLP Helps in Controlling Your Overeating Habit

Weight loss cannot be achieved with NLP, but with NLP, you can change your habits to make it easier to lose weight. What if celery tastes like chocolate? What if you feel better jogging than going to a pub? How easy is it to lose weight? Weight loss is not magic. You simply take in less energy than you emit. NLP for weight loss is also not magic. If you're not sure you're losing weight with NLP, go eat ice cream. However, with NLP, you can achieve weight loss by making the ice cream look unattractive.

Here are some tips to remember when using NLPs as a tool to help you to lose weight:

- An extraordinarily effective device is to "destiny pace" yourself into already having finished the weight reduction. Step into that spot in case you have already reached your weight reduction goal. What mainly will you feel, pay attention to, and notice at that second in time? You enjoy this association, which means searching through your personal eyes.
- I take your recognition and step into the footwear of your children or the individual that loves you the most; whom do you see? What do you want over there? What instance in which you over there giving Weight Loss
- If you're going to search for a suggestion for weight reduction, select a real version of excellence! It is great to discover a person who now no longer handiest claims to have mastery in motivational or training equipment; however, a person who has achieved it OR seems the part.
- How will your fulfilment with finishing your weight reduction aim affect your life?
- How will it affect others around you?
- What are your values? Isn't having a wholesome frame part of dwelling in a life that's actually for your values? Weight loss the usage of NLP will accomplish this.
- Understand the fantastic goal in the back of overeating or transferring too little. If these items have been to deliver you something fantastic, what might that be? For instance, might you be rewarded with comfort? Fun? Freedom? What are a few different methods to gain this over overeating or transferring too little?
- What triggers (anchors) in your surroundings motivate you to eat?

✓ Who is preventing you from finishing your aim? Be honest.

What is the primary step? Do that this week! Using NLP for weight reduction is a number of the great equipment you may use to install your mind! [89]

New Body, New Life

People worldwide have used different types of visualization techniques, meditations, and prayers for centuries. However, visualizations often get bad raps as mysterious things that aren't based on reality or woo. But the truth is that you don't have to be spiritual to benefit from visualization techniques. Psychologists have studied visualizations to understand how they work. And today, everyone, from professional athletes to CEOs, benefits from visualization technology. Let's see what visualization is and why it is important.

Visualization concerns imagining what you want to achieve in the future. As if it was true today. Use all five senses: sight, smell, touch, taste, and hearing. The visualization process tells the subconscious to recognize the ultimate goal you are thinking of. It reminds you regularly. And it trains your brain to react as if the result is true at the moment [90]

Creative visualization is a great tool for weight loss. By visualizing your body as you wish, you let your subconscious mind shape it so that you look like you imagine it. This does not mean that creative visualization will completely change the shape of your body. This means that when you visualize according to the laws of visualization, you will improve your appearance, lose weight, and become more energetic. Manifest and Achievement make your dreams come true with the law of attraction. Discover how to reveal what you want, no matter your current reality. Please use the coupon code *"Imanifest"*. Of course, you also need to change your eating habits. Visualizing the ideal weight motivates you to do something about it. It imprints the image of the ideal body on your subconscious. Next, your subconscious mind acts on your body and shapes it according to your own spiritual image of yourself. However, you also need a healthy diet and exercise. Proper diet and exercise are essential for losing weight, but with the help of creative visualizations, the process can be faster and more enjoyable [91]

Visualization helps you in many ways to lose weight. Here are some ways by which creative imagining helps you:

- ✓ It can program your subconscious to help you lose weight by motivating you to exercise or reducing the amount of food you eat.
- ✓ Creative visualization can guide you to the diet that is most suitable for you.
- ✓ Repeatedly imagining that you are already thin or about to lose weight affects your body's cells, making your body healthier and stronger, and the mentality in your head. Matches the image.

You need to have these important tips while using creative imagining:

- ✓ **Move to smart mode:** You first need to put your mind in a more powerful and highly programmable state of SMART mode. All you need to do is find an image that you can relax easily and relatively quickly.
- ✓ **Make an affirmation:** You can use affirmations to make any change you desire, whether it changes habits, beliefs, or food choices. Break the addiction; or something else. Ensure that the words used in the affirmation are positively focused and present tense (not future tense).
- ✓ **Melt weigh:** There are many ways to imagine weight melting from the body, but I like these images. Watch the excess weight converted into vital energy stored in the body as energy in a much purer form than fat. You save it as invisible, healing life energy.
- ✓ **Create your ideal self:** Now that the fat has melted and turned into energy, direct your inner attention to your ideal self. Imagine your desired shape and how it feels to sit in its perfect shape. Feel the firm skin, firm muscles, flat stomach, and light presence. Upcoming day and month views after imagining everyday scenes, let's look to the future.
- ✓ **Imagine the scenario you want:** See yourself becoming healthier, calmer, more confident, and more desirable. You may want to imagine more success in your business, a more loving relationship, or a healthier boundary.
- ✓ **Magnetize your future:** Imagine your future version becoming a magnet and pulling you in the direction of complete success when you see you in perfect and ideal shape and body months and years later.

- ✓ **Please give me:** Put it back in your body and let yourself charge. Finally, bring that bright image of your future self-back to your body and imagine a super-successful future self that will be you now when you sit there. Feel the new you just created by successfully charging all the cells in your body. And just before you open your eyes, feel and acknowledge that the visualization you just created will change your life forever.
- ✓ **Tell yourself:** I have created my ideal body with the power of my heart. My extra weight melts me easily and effortlessly, allowing me to continue and always succeed in all areas of my life. [92]

Reconditioning Emotions

When you're working hard at the gym and eating well, it can be frustrating if you don't get the results, you want quickly or if the weight loss starts to slow down. At first, you may find that the number on the scale drops quite quickly but starts to slow down after a while, even if you work hard. Muscle weighs more than fat, so if you build muscle, your weight could increase. It is normal, especially in women, to fluctuate up to 10 pounds a month, especially around their time. Try not to use the scale as the primary measure of success. A tape measure is extremely accurate way to track your progress. Don't over-exercise to lose weight faster, as this can lead to burnout and keep you from returning. What you can do? Remember that muscle weighs more than fat; therefore, it might be possible that the weight you think of as fat could be the weight of muscle [93].

In my experience, I have witnessed that people, especially women, feel depressed during their weight loss program, and some also get uncomfortable after getting their desired body. A 2013 study conducted by North Carolina State University researchers found that when one partner loses weight, the relationship suffers. Researchers have found that a partner's weight loss can make a non-diet partner jealous and insecure about the partnership. They also found that when their partner's weight loss goals weren't aligned, the dieting partner became frustrated, feeling that their partner wasn't committed to losing weight [94]

Other studies warn that weight loss can make people feel unwell. A study by Business Insider found that people who lost 5% of their weight in four years were more depressed than those who maintained their weight for the same period. For years, Selby tried many weight-loss plans, but as her pound melted, she felt sick and didn't get better. "The pursuit of weight loss is more harmful than being overweight in itself," said Dr. Linda Bacon, a quasi-nutritionist at the University of California, Davis, and author of Health at Every Size. According to Bacon, people need to stop trusting their bodies to lose weight, which is detrimental to their health. "We have a good regulatory system for eating right, and diets shut down that system," she points out. [95]

Significant weight loss can lead to anger: When others notice such dramatic physical changes, it can cause a bit of resentment or anger. Not all positive statements need to be flattering. It can be difficult to get the approval of others who haven't given time before and are now making positive comments or asking how weight loss was achieved. Now that you've lost weight when learning how to deal emotionally with physical changes (appearance), you can make others feel superficial and superficial just by actively treating one person. Increase. Some people also experienced negative remarks, commenting that they no longer look "healthy." Counselling can also help a person understand that others may have trouble getting used to a physically `new person` or assist in dealing with jealousy [96].

In any weight loss program, anyone can suffer from this emotional rollercoaster. You are highly motivated at one point, but you lose your heart the next moment. So, what should be done now? This question must be in your mind.

Here is the answer:

- ✓ **"Comparison is a thief of joy."** One should try to focus (internally) on oneself without comparing oneself to others. For obese people, dramatic weight loss is primarily about achieving a healthy physical condition. It should not have superficial consequences (which often leads to a continuous state of disappointment).
- ✓ **Losing weight does not have to automatically give way to self-confidence**, and it should not be expected. Being thin makes people who were previously unfamiliar with going out even thinner when they lose a lot of weight. Self-confidence needs to come **"from the inside"** and learn how to deal with the physical changes happening **"from the outside."** Counselling can be very helpful in helping people understand that solving a problem

does not always solve all of their problems. Learning to **"dress"** a new person in a small size also helps to create positive feelings about such dramatic physical changes. It is not uncommon to buy clothes of previous sizes or to wear regular "oversized" comfort clothes. Counselling also helps understand that dramatic physical changes can affect the body's hormonal cycle. This means that depressive symptoms are normal for a person after losing weight. Hormonal imbalances can affect a person's mood, which exacerbates stress, anxiety, and feelings of anxiety.

- ✓ You lose the idea that weight defines a person. **"You are not your weight."** Skinny does not necessarily mean happiness. Losing weight does not have to mean that the weight struggle is over. The pressure to maintain weight can be similarly difficult without proper understanding and care. Psychologically, it can be beneficial for a person to adopt a new label for himself-replace **"fat"** or **"out of shape"** with **"healthy"** and **"energetic."**

- ✓ Think of losing and maintaining a healthy weight as a lifestyle that means a lifelong effort. One can set goals, but the **"journey"** has no real end. Losing weight and maintaining a healthy weight continues every day.

- ✓ People can also benefit better by finding something that makes them happy, feels good about themselves, and makes them healthy. If you have had difficulty travelling before, book a vacation. Learn new hobbies and indulge in worthwhile projects that enrich your life rather than spoil it. It is also advisable to include anything that does not meet these goals in your daily life.

- ✓ No matter how small, we celebrate it when it comes to fruition. Every success is a success that makes you feel good. It will take some time for introspection.

- ✓ Constant thinking about physical activity and calorie management can put a mental strain on a person. Quiet time helps people regain balance and keep negatives away between low points. [97]

You Achieved Your Goal

Unfortunately, many people who lose weight usually end up regaining weight. In fact, only about 20% of dieters who start overweight have succeeded in losing and maintaining weight over the long term. Yet, don't let yourself down. Several scientifically proven ways to lose weight, from exercise to stress management. Once you reach your weight goal, plan a transition period to increase your chances of maintaining weight after a diet. During this time, slowly adjust your lifestyle and observe the effect on your scale. Rapid changes can lead to weight gain. This transitional stage is also a good time to identify and maintain the dietary habits and exercise patterns learned during the diet over the long term. Changing a healthy diet to a healthy lifestyle can help prevent weight gain.

The following strategies can help you to maintain your healthy weight and diet:

- ✓ Regular exercise plays an important role in maintaining weight. Helps burn excess calories and boost metabolism, two factors needed to achieve energy balance. When energy is balanced, you are burning as many calories as you are consuming. As a result, your weight is more likely to remain the same. Studies show that people who do moderate physical activity for at least 200 minutes a week (30 minutes per day) after losing weight are more likely to maintain weight. Increase.
- ✓ In some cases, higher levels of physical activity may be required to maintain a normal weight. One review concludes that one hour of exercise a day is best for those trying to maintain weight loss. It is important to note that exercise is most helpful in maintaining weight when combined with other lifestyle changes, including following a healthy diet.
- ✓ Eating breakfast can help you maintain your weight. Breakfast eaters tend to develop healthy habits overall. For example, do more exercise and consume more fiber and micronutrients. In addition, eating breakfast is one of the most common behaviors reported by people who have succeeded in maintaining weight loss. According to a study, 78% of the 2,959 people who lost 30 pounds (14 kg) in at least a year eat breakfast daily. Breakfast eaters appear to be very successful in maintaining weight loss, but the evidence is mixed. Studies have not shown that skipping breakfast automatically leads to weight gain and poor eating habits. In fact, skipping breakfast may help some people reach their weight loss and weight maintenance goals. This can be one of those that depend on the individual. If you feel eating breakfast will help you reach your goals, please eat it.

However, if you don't like breakfast or aren't hungry in the morning, skipping breakfast doesn't hurt.
- ✓ Regularly stepping on the scale to monitor your weight is a useful tool for maintaining your weight. This is because it can alert you to progress and promote weight management behavior. When you weigh, you may burn fewer calories throughout the day, which helps you maintain weight loss. In one study, people who weighed six days a week averaged 300 calories less per day than those who weighed less often. How often you weigh yourself is an individual choice. Some people find it useful to weigh daily, while others have successfully checked their weight once or twice a week.
- ✓ Loss of muscle mass is a common side effect of weight loss. Muscle loss reduces metabolism, which can limit your ability to maintain weight. This means you burn fewer calories throughout the day. Specific strength training, such as exercise such as weightlifting, helps prevent this muscle loss and maintain or improve metabolic rate. According to a study, people who gain weight after losing weight are more likely to maintain weight by maintaining muscle mass. We recommend doing strength training at least twice a week to get these benefits. For optimal results, the exercise program should target all muscle groups.
- ✓ One habit that often leads to weight gain is eating a healthy diet on weekdays and having an affair on weekends. This spirit often leads people to eat junk food, which can offset weight maintenance efforts. When it becomes a normal habit, you can gain more weight than you initially lost. Or according to studies, people who follow a consistent dietary pattern throughout the week are more likely to lose weight in the long run. According to one study, those who gained flexibility over the weekend are almost twice as likely to keep their weight within 5 pounds (2.2 kg) in a year while maintaining weekly consistency.
- ✓ Drinking water helps maintain weight for several reasons. For beginners, drinking a glass or two before meals may increase satiety and help reduce calorie intake. In one study, people who drank water before meals had 13% lower caloric intake than participants who did not drink water. In addition, drinking water has been shown to slightly increase the number of calories burned throughout the day.

- ✓ Getting enough sleep has a big impact on weight management. In fact, sleep deprivation appears to be a major risk factor for weight gain in adults and can interfere with weight maintenance. This is because lack of sleep raises the level of ghrelin, known as the hunger hormone, to increase appetite. In addition, people who lack sleep tend to have lower levels of leptin, a hormone required for appetite control. In addition, people who sleep only for a short time are simply tired, discouraging them from exercising and choosing a healthy diet. If you're not getting enough sleep, find a way to adjust your sleep habits. At least 7 hours of sleep at night is best for weight management and overall health.

These are some helpful tips that can help you to maintain your weight. Keep in mind that getting to succeed is a normal thing, but sustaining that success is more important. A lot of people end up regaining weight. This is sad because all their struggles are lost within a few days. Therefore, these tips can help you.[98]

CHAPTER #7 - TECHNIQUES TO APPLY

We have descrive everything regarding your weight loss program. You must be well aware of your health. The main objective of this chapter is to give you brief but comprehensive details about the food you eat and what exercise you do. This chapter still helps even if you are not obese and overweight is not your problem, this chapter still helps you. I would talk about the foods that are good for your health and not. That is true that everything you eat provides you nutrition. For the normal functioning of our body, we need fat, protein, vitamins, minerals, etc., to sustain our life.

Excess to anything, including water, is dangerous. Therefore, it is advised that there should be a variety of meals every day so that we could get a "moderate" amount. Hence, for me, there is no such thing as bad food. The concept is that meals are fuel that each meal will nourish your body, and that variant and moderation are vital keys to nourishing the frame well. We ought to alternate our language around meals to interrupt unfastened from this mentality. Pay interest to whether or not descriptions of meals are fantastic or negative. Counteract the numerous messages from the media by pronouncing in response, *"Food is fuel!"* Remember that regardless of what you're eating, it's far offering vitamins on your frame. All meals are good meals.

As I said, there is no bad meal. Why do people usually declare some foods as harmful or bad? The answer to this question is simple. They, in reality, do not call the food bad; it's the way of eating which makes it a health hazard. Therefore, I will show you some ways which make every food notorious and delicious. Moreover, you will also get simple food plans. No matter the category you fall in, they would be good for toddlers to adults.

Good Foods and Bad Foods

As a physical coach, I will always encourage you to make nutritious choices to benefit your overall body and health. While there are no "bad" foods, certain foods do not provide as many benefits to the body as others. Some foods have ingredients that are not nutritious for the body, like Tran's fats and artificial additives. But that does not mean we should form strict and rigid rules avoiding those foods for the rest of our life or attaching morality to them. You are not a better person if you eat more nutritious food, and you are not worse if you eat something less nutritious. Life is not perfect and involves making choices considering your circumstances, tastes and preferences.

When we label foods as "good" or "bad," we are giving that meal too much control and power, which has the potential to lead to disordered eating. Restricting ourselves from food can ultimately backfire and lead to a binge-restrict cycle that is unhealthy for your physical body, mental health, and wellbeing. Designating certain foods as bad can also lead to unnecessary stress and preoccupation with these items.

Therefore, I would advise you to listen to your body; if you are craving food, then know its okay to eat your favorite foods in moderation without guilt or judgment. Every meal does not have to be the perfect, most nutritious meal of your life. One meal, snack, or food does not define your nutrition status or self-worth. [99]

However, I will tell you about some eatables. Remember that no food is bad as food is the body's fuel. It's the excess of meal which makes it harmful.

Following foods, you should eat moderately and not regularly:

- ✓ Whole eggs
- ✓ Leafy greens
- ✓ Salmon
- ✓ Cruciferous vegetables
- ✓ Chicken breast and some lean meats
- ✓ Potatoes and other root vegetables
- ✓ Tuna
- ✓ Beans and legumes
- ✓ Soups
- ✓ Cottage cheese
- ✓ Avocados
- ✓ Nuts

- ✓ Whole grains
- ✓ Chili pepper
- ✓ Fruit
- ✓ Grapefruit
- ✓ Chia seeds
- ✓ Full fat (whole) Greek yoghurt [100]

Good and Bad Ways of Eating

We have already discussed bad eating habits (see chapter 1). As I said above, the food is not bad; rather, how you eat it makes it good or bad. Let's just take a simple example. If you are eating meat, a great protein source, mindless and continuous eating can lead to serious outcomes like meat addiction. And the most prominent one is obesity.

In this section, I will tell you some ways to make anything you eat nutritiously.:

- ✓ Chew your meals for as a minimum of 10 seconds earlier than swallowing.
- ✓ Pack a self-made lunch/breakfast for school, and ensure it consists of a nutritious snack (e.g., reduce fruits, simple or oat biscuits).
- ✓ Eat slowly; it takes a couple of minutes for the mind to comprehend the belly is full.
- ✓ Drink a pitcher of water or have a bowl of soup to keep away from overeating.
- ✓ Schedule your meal times/devour on time.
- ✓ Get greater fire (e.g., entire grains and legumes).
- ✓ Eat smaller meal portions.
- ✓ Drink greater water.
- ✓ Eat in moderation
- ✓ Eat only when you are starving
- ✓ Never skip your breakfast
- ✓ Eat plenty of meals kinds meal.
- ✓ Choose ingredients that can be steamed, braised, or grilled in preference to deep-fried [101]

Best Food Plan

Diets aren't only for weight loss. While converting your food regimen may be one of the unique approaches to losing weight, it could also be a gateway to enhancing your habits, focusing on your fitness, and maintaining a greater energetic lifestyle. Yet the sheer variety of to-be-had food regimen plans may make it tough to start.

Different diets can be greater suitable, sustainable, and powerful for extraordinary people. Some diets' purpose is to decrease your urge for food to lessen your meal consumption. In contrast, others advocate proscribing your consumption of energy and both carbs and fat. Some are more conscious of positive consuming styles and lifestyle changes in preference to proscribing positive foods. What's greater, many provide fitness blessings that pass past weight loss. [102]

It's important to keep a few factors in mind when selecting the best meal plan for yourself.

- ✓ For starters, be sure to consider your personal needs and preferences. While some people may enjoy structured diet programs, others might prefer plans that are a bit more flexible. Certain meal plans may also require more time and effort than others, which can be an important consideration for women who might not want to measure portion sizes or track their food intake.
- ✓ Avoid diets that eliminate entire food groups or are very restrictive. These meal plans are more difficult to follow for longer, but they can also make it much more difficult to get all the required nutrients.
- ✓ Finally, be sure to talk with a healthcare professional before making any changes to your diet. This is very important if you have health issues or are taking medications [103].

Eating plans help you to balance your diet. They help you target your meal intake and have an important role in it.

Following are some tips that can aid you in making a perfect weekly eating plan:

Step 1: Make a Menu First

Reflect on consideration on your technique for meal planning — do you:

- ✓ Want to make a weekly or a month-to-month plan? Prefer to put together food beforehand of time, simply earlier than the meal or a mixture of both?
- ✓ Want to choose an afternoon to prepare dinner
- ✓ Food for the week or a month that you could shop with inside the freezer?
- ✓ Need to consider any unique vitamin wish for yourself or your circle of relatives?
- ✓ Next, both on a sheet of paper, on your smartphone, or on the computer, create your menu:
- ✓ Take a minute to examine how to prepare a healthful meal and ensure you are becoming the proper quantity for every meal group.
- ✓ Flip through cookbooks or online websites and discover recipes that appear properly. Evaluate the extent of cooking talent required to make the recipe. Do you have those skills? If not, are you up for the challenge? Also, ensure that you have any unique cooking utensils or pans for the recipe.
- ✓ Check in together along with your own circle of relatives approximately, their schedules, and meal preferences. Weigh the elements as you prepare your menu.
- ✓ Think about the weather. Hearty soups and stews are perfect for a chilly winter's night. A salad with lean protein could make an ideal entrée on a warm summertime season day. If packing lunches, ensure that any perishables may be saved in a fridge or an insulated bag with an ice pack.
- ✓ Find out what substances you have already got on hand. It is fine to always rotate foodstuffs instead of shopping them for lengthy intervals. So, try and expand the gadgets which you have on hand. You'll additionally store money!
- ✓ Check out the income at your neighborhood supermarkets. Sometimes a reduced rate can permit you to deal with yourself and your circle of relatives to an amazing meal.
- ✓ Aim for a range in food, but don't experience like each day should be different. Eating oatmeal or low-fat yoghurt with berries every week is okay for breakfast. The equal is going for lunch; choose some alternatives and rotate them weekly. Jot down breakfast, lunch, and dinner alternatives. And, don't overlook snacks.
- ✓ Think about the way to deal with leftovers. Might you serve them once more that week or freeze them for any other week? Consider meal safety,

as refrigerated leftovers must be used up for 3 to 4 days or frozen for later use.
- ✓ Run the menu with the aid of using others in your household. Does its appearance properly to them? Make any modifications wished.
- ✓ During the week, preserve notes approximately how nicely the menu worked. These notes can remind you of approaches to enhance your recipes and menu. [104]

Step 2: Stock Your Pantry and Freezer with the Five Food Groups

To begin meal planning, take time to inventory the fundamentals. This consists of healthful meals which you want to consume and prepare. The lists underneath offers pantry and freezer objects to inventory up on from the 5 meal groups. Circle the objects you need to inventory in your pantry and freezer. Plus, upload different objects based on your non-public fitness wishes and meal preferences.

Five Food Groups Pantry List

- ✓ **Vegetables**: Keep numerous canned tomatoes in inventory (diced, crushed, whole, stewed). Use them in soups, stews, sauces, casseroles, and more! Also, select a bottle of your preferred spaghetti sauce. Dried mushrooms are other extraordinary pantry objects because they can upload the intensity of taste to your meals.
- ✓ **Fruits**: Raisins, dried cranberries, dried apricots, and different dried fruits; the end result are loaded with nutritional fiber. They upload a punch of taste to your morning breakfast, noon salad, and dinner grains.
- ✓ **Milk and Dairy Products**: Dried milk is an extraordinary backup object to have on inventory. You can use it for your espresso or tea. Boxed milk is likewise to be had in single-serving applications and is an extraordinary object for lunch boxes. In cans within the baking aisle, Evaporated milk may be substituted for liquid milk in full recipes.
- ✓ **Protein Foods**: Stock up on canned or dried lentils, black, pinto, cannellini, garbanzo, and kidney beans. These legumes are an excellent supply of protein. Toss cooked beans in salads, soups, stews, and different dishes.

Canned tuna, anchovies, and sardines are a pantry must — they're quick to feature protein, healthful fat, and taste to meals.

- ✓ **Grains**: Keep a stash of oatmeal, buckwheat, and different whole-grain cereals withinside the pantry. Add nuts and clean berries to those warm cereals for an additional increase. Barley, farro, quinoa, and different grains offer staples for healthful meals. Also, preserve numerous rice on hand — lengthy grain, short grain, basmati, and brown rice. Spaghetti, ziti, penne, and different pasta are extraordinary for an easy, brief, and filling own circle of relatives. Give yourself an additional vitamin increase by shopping for whole-grain pasta or attempting pasta crafted from legumes.

Also, inventory is up on:

- ✓ **Condiments**: Ketchup, mustard, and pleasure may be saved within the pantry until they're opened. Once you open them, preserve them with inside the fridge.
- ✓ **Oil and vinegar:** Extra-virgin olive oil is a versatile, heart-healthful option. Other oils, including peanut, walnut, and sesame, upload a burst of taste to meals. Pick up unique forms of vinegar, including cider, white and balsamic. Each imparts a completely unique taste to your recipes.
- ✓ **Stock**: Vegetable, hen, and red meat inventory are the fundamentals of many recipes. Opt for the ones that are low-sodium or comprise no delivered salt.
- ✓ **Herbs and spices:** Pick up small bins of floor herbs and spices. In that manner, they're as clean as viable while you operate them.
- ✓ **Flax and different seeds:** Flax and chia seeds are the supply of protein, fibre, and omega-three fatty acids. Add them to cereal, salads, sauces, and home-baked goods. If you purchase whole flaxseed, ensure you grind it up earlier than ingesting so your frame can soak up the vitamins.

Five Food Groups Freezer List

To ensure you don't save meals past freshness, place dates at the applications earlier than storing them within the freezer. And use the oldest first.

- ✓ **Vegetables:** Pick up a number of your favorite frozen veggies. These are a top-notch supply of vitamins, minerals, and different vitamins because the flash-freezing manner locks with inside the nutrients. Look for containers without sodium. And, at the same time as you're with inside the produce aisle, clutch a few pure herbs. When you get home, fill ice dice trays with chopped herbs, pinnacle off the herbs with boiling water, and punctiliously vicinity the freezer. Add those herbal cubes for a punch of freshness to your meals.

- ✓ **Fruits:** Stash frozen berries and different culmination withinside the freezer. They are a top-notch manner to feature nutrients in a morning smoothie.
- ✓ **Milk and Dairy Products:** Freeze Parmesan and pre-shredded cheeses — toss them into soups, stews, and pasta dishes. Low-fat, frozen yoghurt may be a quick dessert for a unique occasion.
- ✓ **Protein Foods:** Stock up on salmon and different fatty fishes to ensure you're prepared and get the right of entry to wholesome fats. Frozen lean meats and fowl additionally save properly withinside the freezer. One tip: make certain you circulate it to the fridge sooner or later than cooking to provide an okay time for defrosting. Keep a whole lot of nuts withinside the freezer. This facilitates save you them from spoiling. Add them to bloodless cereal, salads, warm grains, and dishes.
- ✓ **Grains:** Whole-grain corn tortillas freeze properly and may be used for quick breakfasts, lunches, or dinners. Can't consume that loaf of bread sufficient simultaneously as it's far clean? Make it an addiction to freeze a part of the loaf and defrost slices as you want them. [105]

Step 3: Keep a Running Grocery List

In a convenient place, keep a pad and pen and write them down on the list as you use up grocery items. This way, you don't have to worry about forgetting anything when you hit the supermarket. Or use an app for that.

Diet Plans for Men

- ✓ **High protein diets:** Diets excessive in protein may also sell weight reduction and assist you to hold a healthful frame of weight over time
- ✓ **The Mediterranean Diet:** Research shows that the Mediterranean weight loss program promotes weight reduction and protects against coronary heart disorder and different fitness situations.

- ✓ **Whole meals, plant-primarily based diet:** WFPB diets emphasize complete plant meals. However, they will consist of small quantities of animal products. Such diets may also enhance men's fitness and inspire weight reduction.
- ✓ **Low carb diets:** Research has cited that low carb diets may also enhance weight reduction. Choosing a milder model in carbs is probably higher for a long-time period of weight maintenance.
- ✓ **High fiber diets:** Eating greater fiber may also assist guys in attaining and holding a healthful frame weight, in addition to lessening disorder risk.
- ✓ **Diets that concentrate on power and nutrient density:** Eating greater low-calorie, nutrient-dense meals can assist guys in attaining and holding a healthful frame weight.
- ✓ **The paleo weight loss program:** The paleo weight loss program may also assist guys in losing extra frame fats and enhancing sure markers of metabolic fitness, blood pressure, triglycerides, and blood sugar levels.
- ✓ **The MIND weight loss program:** The MIND weight loss program combines factors of the Mediterranean and DASH diets to inspire healthful, nutrient-dense meals that sell mind fitness. It additionally makes a high-quality desire for weight management.
- ✓ **Intermittent energy restriction (IER)** IER may also cause weight reduction and different components of men's fitness.
- ✓ **Vegetarian diets:** Vegetarian diets excessive in nutrient-dense plant meals may also cause decreased calorie consumption and assist guys in losing extra frame fats. [106]

Diet Plans for Women

Nutrient-rich foods provide energy for women's busy lives and help to reduce the risk of disease. **<u>A healthy eating plan regularly includes:</u>**

- ✓ At least three ounce-equivalents of whole grains such as whole-grain bread, whole-wheat cereal flakes, whole-wheat pasta, bulgur, quinoa, brown rice, or oats.
- ✓ Three servings of low-fat or fat-free dairy products, including milk, yoghurt or cheese, or calcium-fortified soymilk. (Non-dairy sources of

calcium for people who do not consume dairy products include calcium-fortified foods and beverages, canned fish, and some leafy greens.)
- ✓ Five to 5-and-a-half ounce-equivalents of protein foods such as lean meat, poultry, seafood, eggs, beans, lentils, tofu, nuts, and seeds.
- ✓ Half to two cups of fresh, frozen, canned, or dried fruits without added sugars.
- ✓ Two to two-and-a-half cups of colorful vegetables — fresh, frozen, or canned without added salt [107]

Diet plan for kids

Nutrition for children is primarily based totally on the very ideas of vitamins for adults. Everyone desires identical forms of vitamins, including vitamins, minerals, carbohydrates, protein, and fats. Children, however, want special quantities of particular vitamins at certain ages. So, what's the good system to boost your toddler's increase and development? Check out those fundamental vitamins for girls and boys at numerous ages.

Consider those nutrient-dense meals:

- ✓ **Protein:** Choose seafood, lean meat and hen, eggs, beans, peas, soy products, and unsalted nuts and seeds.
- ✓ **Fruits:** Encourage your toddler to devour a lot of fresh, canned, frozen, or dried culmination — as opposed to fruit juice. If your toddler liquids juice, ensure it is a hundred per cent juice without delivered sugars and restrictions on their servings. Look for canned fruit that asserts it is mild or packed in its very own juice, which means it is low in delivered sugar. Remember that one-region cup of dried fruit counts as one cup-equal fruit. When fed on in excess, dried culmination can contribute to greater energy.
- ✓ **Vegetables:** Serve a lot of fresh, canned, frozen, or dried greens. Aim to offer a lot of greens, darkish green, pink and orange, beans and peas, starchy, and others every week. When deciding on canned or frozen greens, search for alternatives with decreases in sodium.

- ✓ **Grains:** Choose complete grains, including complete-wheat bread, oatmeal, popcorn, quinoa, or brown or wild rice. Limit subtle grains, which include white bread, pasta, and rice.
- ✓ **Dairy:** Encourage your toddler to devour and drink fats-unfastened or low-fat dairy products, including milk, yoghurt, cheese, or fortified soy beverages.

Aim to restrict your toddler's energy from:

- ✓ **Added sugar:** Limit delivered sugars. Naturally, going on sugars, which includes the ones in fruit and milk, aren't delivered sugars. Examples of delivered sugars include brown sugar, corn sweetener, corn syrup, honey, and others. Check vitamins labels. Choose cereals with minimum delivered sugars. Avoid liquids with delivered sugars, including soda, sports activities, and power liquids.
- ✓ **Saturated and trans-fat:** Limit saturated fat — fat that particularly comes from animal sources of food, which includes red meat, hen, and full-fat dairy products. Look for approaches to update saturated fat with vegetable and nut oils, which give important fatty acids and nutrients. Healthier fat is also clearly found in olives, nuts, avocados, and seafood. Limit trans-fat via way of means of heading off meals that include in part hydrogenated oil.
- ✓ **Sodium:** Most youngsters within the U.S. have excessive sodium in their daily diets. Encourage snacking on culmination and greens as opposed to chips and cookies. Check vitamin labels and search for products low in sodium. [108]

Diet plan for adults

A wholesome weight-reduction plan consists of the following:

- ✓ Fruit, veggies, legumes (e.g., lentils and beans), nuts, and entire grains (e.g., unprocessed maize, millet, oats, wheat, and brown rice).
- ✓ At least four hundred grams (i.e., 5 portions) of fruit and veggies consistent with the day, except for potatoes, candy potatoes, cassava, and different starchy roots.

- ✓ Less than 10% of total energy consumption from unfastened sugars equal to 50 g (or approximately 12 stage teaspoons) for someone of healthy body weight ingesting approximately 2000 energy consistent with day, however preferably is much less than five% of general power consumption for added fitness benefits. Free sugars are all sugars delivered to meals or liquids through the manufacturer, prepare dinner, or consumer, in addition to sugars found in honey, syrups, fruit juices, and fruit juice concentrates.
- ✓ Less than 30% of general power consumption is from fat. Unsaturated fat (determined in fish, avocado, and nuts, and in sunflower, soybean, canola, and olive oils) leads to saturated fat (determined in fatty meat, butter, palm, and coconut oil, cream, cheese, ghee, and lard) and trans-fat of all kinds, which includes each industrially-produced trans-fat (determined in baked and fried meals, and pre-packaged snacks and meals, which include frozen pizza, pies, cookies, biscuits, wafers, and cooking oils and spreads) and ruminant trans-fat (determined in meat and dairy meals from ruminant animals, which include cows, sheep, goats, and camels). It is recommended that saturated fat consumption be decreased to less than 10% of general power consumption and trans-fat to much less than 1% of general power consumption. In particular, industrially-produced trans-fat isn't a part of a wholesome weight-reduction plan and must be avoided. Less than five g of salt (equal to approximately one teaspoon) is consistent daily. Salt needs to be iodized. [109]

TELL ME ABOUT YOU

Do you want to continue overeating? Or do you want to be free? If you feel confused, make your decision only after reading the book and putting into practice everything it advices. "The fear of giving up doing something, of taking risks by leaving what we know and changing things is inherent in all of us". I tried to explain to Margaret when she confided her uncertainty. "However, there comes a time when you realize that you can no longer go on as you always have, that you need to change course that you have to take the risk because there is a higher stake." The same is for you.

What pushed you to be here, to hold this book in your hands and read it?

_____

_____

_____

Well, why are you reading this?

_____

_____

What do you mean? Explain better.

_____

_____

Well, ultimately are you reading this because...?

_____

_____

It seems like the same question repeated, I know. But it is not. Or rather, it is partly in order to elaborate a more useful to you answer.

> **I'll give you an example:**
>
> Why are you reading this book?
>
> Because they recommended it to me.
>
> What do you mean? Explain better...
>
> Because I eat too much and I would like to stop. I have tried many times in vain.
>
> Well, ultimately are reading you this because...?
>
> I want to be fit and be able to eat regularly.

I don't want to condition your answer with this example. I have included it just to make it clearer that, when we answer a question, we are unlikely to be honest at the first answer, especially with ourselves and if the topic is to quit smoking. But usually, after three questions, the true and profound motivation comes out, without excuses or resistance, or in any case you get close to the truth. I want you to be honest with yourself.

<u>*Write down what you feel, what and how you would like it to be.*</u>

What would you *want* to happen reading this book?

_____

_____

Now, that you have given the answer, convince me that what you have written is true, that it is useful to you. What are the reasons for your answer?

> **I'll give you an example:**
>
> I want to get rid of obesity and fat forever. I am tired from all the times I have tried to in vain, and I feel unmotivated.
>
> I would like to be free from my food addition and I would like to succeed this time.
>
> What motivations support this goal of yours?
>
> - I have several problems with the opposite sex.
>
> - I am not a good example for my children.
>
> - I get tired very often.
>
> - I want to improve my fitness.

Answer:

_____

_____

List of reasons in support of the answer:

_____

_____

Now, for each of the reasons you have filled in, be specific and expand what you have written by asking yourself the **"reason why"**.

> **Example:** *I am not a good example for my children.*
>
> Why? What are the behaviours, thoughts and emotions that make you say this?

I feel guilty when I say that in life you must be strong and committed, while I am feeling weak and incapable, without willpower!

This is just an example, it may not concern you, but you certainly also have good reasons and contradictions in terms of values. The more the motivations are specific and oriented towards a positive dimension, the more powerful, and constructive and closer they are to our deepest values. Instinctively answer the questions I ask you: the more often you think, the worse it is. Put your stomach and heart in front of reasoning. The answers will serve as a map to better orient you in the depths of your mind. Write as much as you can. The clearer and more detailed you are, the sooner you free yourself.

Talk to your stimulus

> **Any question or doubt that comes to your mind, I propose another very powerful exercise**
>
> If you want to overeating with junk food, the first thing to do is... don't smoke it! Of course, this is obvious, you will tell me. But now I'm going to teach you to familiarize yourself with a technique that will make a difference. **I'll let you talk to the symptom!**
>
> 1. Accept the stimulus. Remember that the symptom always has something to tell you. What comes from us always has a positive function. Nothing that comes to us is born with the intention of harming us.

2. Talk to "him". Now, imagine having in front of you, sitting on a chair, Mr. Stimulus, and have a chat with him. Follow the questions and address them to your stimulus as if he were sitting in front of you, in flesh and blood. Then give him time to respond. With a little patience and training you will get the first results. I know, it's not a walk in the park, but this exercise, with a little commitment, has helped many of the people I followed in coaching because it provides a key to reframe the problems and give them a new meaning.

Let's see the exercise step by step:

1. Ask your stimulus: "Do you want to talk to me?" Yes/No? If he answers No, give him some time. He must trust you after you have neglected him for too long. Let him understand that it is important to you.

2. Say, "I accept you; you are part of me. Thanks for existing, I know you want my good".

3. Ask, "What is your positive function?" Make it specific. What it protects you from, why it does it, etc. Give him time, if he doesn't answer, repeat the question.

4. Ask, "What can I do to have your intention respected and propel me towards wellness?"

If you cannot answer immediately, do not be discouraged! It is difficult to question who we are, what we want and why, yet it is necessary to bring out the best in ourselves. Trust yourself and your feelings, stay anchored to the answers. Engage in answering, give yourself permission to do so. The answers may not arrive immediately but use the strategy of repeating the questions as soon as you can. You will hear the answer emerge and tell you the truth.

REVIEW THIS BOOK

I trust all is to your satisfaction.

Thank you for having got this far! I hope it was to your taste. I would be extremely grateful if you would take 1 minute of your time to leave a review on Amazon about **HOW TO STOP OVEREATING AND LOSE WEIGHT EASILY!**

Go to www.bookyourdestiny.com

CONCLUSION

You have come down this long book, and I am sure you may have learnt something new. As a physical trainer, I wish that you get the desired figure you have always wanted. For most obese, losing weight seems like a big mountain to climb. They have developed eating as their second nature. They also ride on an emotional rollercoaster. Sometimes, they are motivated, and in the next moment, they lose their heart.

Most importantly, the first and the most difficult barrier is the barrier of mind. If you have overcome it, congratulations! You are among those who can face the hardships of life. Losing weight itself feels impossible when you have been suffering from binge eating. Most the coaches remain in the triangle of workout, diet and psychology when it comes to losing weight. However, I also talked about Neuro-Linguistic Programming, which is an effective tool not for losing weight but for keeping you on track. Visualization also helps you stay on track, as not being able to see desired results in a few days can be fed you up.

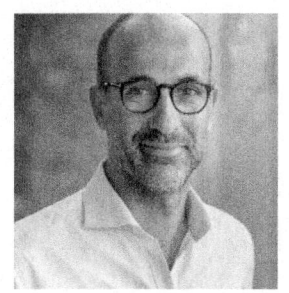

The Author

Han Carrel (1978) is a *coach*. He has been working in the field of personal growth for over sixteen years. With an always attentive look at the most innovative methods of improvement, effective communication and coaching for psychophysical well-being.

REFERENCES

1. Fabricatore, Anthony N., and Thomas A. Wadden. "Psychological aspects of obesity." Clinics in dermatology 22.4 (2004): 332-337.

2. Masheb, Robin M., et al. "Pain and emotional eating: further investigation of the Yale Emotional Overeating Questionnaire in weight loss seeking patients." Journal of Behavioral Medicine 43.3 (2020): 479-486

3. Smith, Trenton G. "Reconciling psychology with economics: Obesity, behavioral biology, and rational overeating." Journal of Bioeconomics 11.3 (2009): 249-282.

4. https://www.foundationsrecoverynetwork.com/what-are-narcotics-and-why-are-they-addictive/

5. Nicola Davis, The Guardian, "Is Sugar Really Addictive as Cocaine?", 2017

6. Van Opstal, A. M., et al. "Dietary sugars and non-caloric sweeteners elicit different homeostatic and hedonic responses in the brain." Nutrition 60 (2019): 80-86.

7. https://www.psychiatry.org/patients-families/eating-disorders/what-are-eating-disorders

8. Mayo Clinic, "Binge-Eating Disorder", 2018

9. https://www.psychiatry.org/patients-families/eating-disorders/what-are-eating-disorders

10. Randy Fang, "Prevalence of Eating Disorders in Men versus Women", 2010

11. Cao, Jay J. "Effects of obesity on bone metabolism." Journal of orthopaedic surgery and research 6.1 (2011): 1-7.

12. Murugan, A. T., and G. Sharma. "Obesity and respiratory diseases." Chronic respiratory disease 5.4 (2008): 233-242.

13. Pasquali, R., A. Gambineri, and U. Pagotto. "The impact of obesity on reproduction in women with polycystic ovary syndrome." BJOG: An International Journal of Obstetrics & Gynaecology 113.10 (2006): 1148-1159.

14. Du Plessis, Stefan S., et al. "The effect of obesity on sperm disorders and male infertility." Nature Reviews Urology 7.3 (2010): 153-161.

15. Poirier, Paul, and Robert H. Eckel. "Obesity and cardiovascular disease." Current atherosclerosis reports 4.6 (2002): 448-453.

16. Moore, Catherine F., et al. "Pathological overeating: emerging evidence for a compulsivity construct." Neuropsychopharmacology 42.7 (2017): 1375-1389.

17. Samantha Bothwell, "Understanding Compulsive Eating Disorder: Symptoms, Causes, & Treatment"

18. Jennifer Rainey Marquiz, "Compulsive Overeating and How to Stop It?", 2022

19. Macht, Michael, and Gwenda Simons. "Emotional eating." Emotion regulation and well-being. Springer, New York, NY, 2011. 281-295.

20. Moore, Catherine F., et al. "Pathological overeating: emerging evidence for a compulsivity construct." Neuropsychopharmacology 42.7 (2017): 1375-1389.

21. French, Simone A., and Robert W. Jeffery. "Consequences of dieting to lose weight: effects on physical and mental health." Health Psychology 13.3 (1994): 195.

22. Kenney, Erica, and Koushik Adhikari. "Recent developments in identifying and quantifying emotions during food consumption." Journal of the Science of Food and Agriculture 96.11 (2016): 3627-3630.

23. Mental Health Foundation, "Diet and Mental Health", 2022

24. Biron Team, "The harmful effects of salts on your health", 2021

25. Cleveland Clinic, "How Salt Can Impact Your Blood Pressure, Heart and Kidneys", 2020

26. National Kidney Foundation, "Sugar and Your Kidneys", 2017

27. James Januzzi, Nasrien Ibrahim, "Heart Failure and Salt-The Great Debate", 2018

28. Harvard Medical School, "The Sweet Danger of Sugar", 2022

29. Darren Wee, "10 Clever Things Fast Food Chains Do To Attract Customers", 2016

30. Jay Zagorsky, "Will Regulating Fast Food Really Help Poor People?", 2017

31. https://budgetbranders.com/fast-food-statistics/

32. Melissa Healy, "By 2030, nearly half of U.S. adults will be obese, experts predict", 2019

33. https://www.futurity.org/trump-fast-food-2251772/

34. https://www.mindtools.com/pages/article/newTCS_95.htm

35. Brenda Goodman, Jennifer Casarella, "Food Addiction," 2020

36. Kris Gunnars, "8 Common Symptoms of Food Addiction", 2019

37. Melissa Dahl, "Can eating too much make your stomach burst?", 2011

38. Mayo Clinic, "Binge-Eating Disorder", 2018

39. Kugelmann, Robert. "Willpower." Theory & Psychology 23.4 (2013): 479-498.

40. https://portal.peopleonehealth.com/HealthyLiving/Health/All/WriteYourVisionStatementforWeightLoss

41. Shari Broder, "12 Common Excuses for Overeating and Why They're Lies", 2016

42. Lauren Brown, "39 Ways to Turn Off the Chatter in Your Head About Food", 2020

43. Lauren Brown, "39 Ways to Turn Off the Chatter in Your Head About Food", 2020

44. https://www.headspace.com/meditation/weight-loss

45. Lauren Brown, "39 Ways to Turn Off the Chatter in Your Head About Food", 2020

46. https://online.maryville.edu/blog/self-empowerment/

47. https://mccartyweightloss.com/how-weight-loss-can-boost-your-energy-self-esteem/

48. https://www.takingcharge.csh.umn.edu/how-does-food-impact-health

49. https://www.sahealth.sa.gov.au/wps/wcm/connect/public+content/sa+health+internet/healthy+living/is+your+health+at+risk/the+risks+of+poor+nutrition

50. Wansink, Brian. "From mindless eating to mindlessly eating better." Physiology & behavior 100.5 (2010): 454-463.

51. Gallant, Annette, Jennifer Lundgren, and Vicky Drapeau. "Nutritional aspects of late eating and night eating." Current obesity reports 3.1 (2014): 101-107.

52. Rani, Rekha, Chetan N. Dharaiya, and Bhopal Singh. "Importance of not skipping breakfast: A review." International Journal of Food Science & Technology 56.1 (2021): 28-38.

53. Nora Belblidia, "Negative Emotions Cause Stronger Appetite Responses in Emotional Eaters", 2020

54. https://www.everydayhealth.com/diet-and-nutrition-pictures/bad-eating-habits-and-how-to-break-them.aspx

55. https://www.mensjournal.com/health-fitness/five-reasons-a-weight-loss-coach-may-be-best-for-you/

56. https://www.fitmotherproject.com/best-exercises-to-lose-weight/

57. https://www.healthline.com/health/fitness/benefits-of-kettle-bell-swings#how-to-do-one

58. Paige Waehner, "How to do mountain climbers-Proper form, variations and common mistakes", 2021

59. https://gethealthyu.com/exercise/renegade-rows/

60. Christa Sagoba, "How to do squats correctly to make the most of the move", 2020

61. Kimberly Dawn Neumann, Maggie Seaver, "Here's how to do squats properly, safely and effectively all the time", 2022

62. Katz, Jack. How emotions work. University of Chicago Press, 1999, 1

63. Tony Ambush, "Emotional Components of Weight Loss." 2016

64. Malia Frey, Rachel Goldman, "How to Overcome 5 Psychological Blocks to Weight Loss", 2021

65. https://www.cdc.gov/healthyweight/physical_activity/index.html

66. Katey Davidson, "Is diet or exercise more important for your health", 2021

67. Arnaud Chiolero, David Faeh, Fred Paccaud, Jacques Cornuz, Consequences of smoking for body weight, body fat distribution, and insulin resistance, *The American Journal of Clinical Nutrition*, Volume 87, Issue 4, April 2008, Pages 801–809

68. Ryan Raman, "The 9 Best Diet Plans for Your Overall Health", 2022

69. Ryan Raman, "The 9 Best Diet Plans for Your Overall Health", 2022

70. https://www.mayoclinic.org/healthy-lifestyle/nutrition-and-healthy-eating/in-depth/dash-diet/art-20048456

71. Cleveland Clinic, "What is the Flexitarian diet?", 2021

72. Keith Pearson, "The MIND Diet: A Detailed Guide for Beginners", 2017

73. Ryan Raman, "The 9 Best Diet Plans for Your Overall Health", 2022

74. https://www.mayoclinic.org/healthy-lifestyle/nutrition-and-healthy-eating/expert-answers/intermittent-fasting/faq-20441303

75. Rachel Link, "Volumetrics Diet Review", 2020

76. Kameshwari Kovvli, "Top 10 fat burning sports to lose weight", 2017

77. https://www.asics.com/gb/en-gb/running-advice/how-to-lose-belly-fat-by-running/

78. https://www.sportsver.com/is-racquetball-a-good-workout-weight-loss-activity/

79. https://www.livestrong.com/article/542736-does-soccer-make-you-lose-weight/

80. Jacob Stutsman, "Can You Lose Weight by Playing Basketball?", 2021

81. https://fitboxmethod.com/3-ways-boxing-helps-you-lose-weight-fast/

82. Jennifer Larson, Daniel Bubins, "Biking for Weight Loss: 4 Effective Strategies to Try", 2020

83. Liz Burton Hughes, "Neuro Linguistic Programming- A Beginners Guide", 2015

84. Wendy Boring-Bey, "The Visualization Definition and How it Transforms Your Life", 2021

85. https://www.tonyrobbins.com/leadership-impact/nlp-techniques/

86. https://ellymcguinness.com/blog/nlp-for-weight-loss/

87. Timothy J. Legg, "What is NLP and What is Used For?", 2017

88. https://ellymcguinness.com/blog/nlp-for-weight-loss/

89. Nicole Schneider, "10 Tips: How to Use NLP for Weight Loss", 2014

90. Kristine Moe, "5 Visualization Techniques to Help You Reach You Reach our Goals", 2021

91. https://www.successconsciousness.com/blog/creative-visualization/lose-weight-with-creative-visualization/

92. Jon Gabriel, *"7 Easy Steps to Visualize Your Weight Loss"*, 2016

93. https://www.nuffieldhealth.com/article/the-emotional-rollercoaster-of-weight-loss

94. https://www.healthline.com/health/losing-weight-and-relationships

95. https://www.healthline.com/health/losing-weight-and-relationships

96. https://www.mymed.com/diseases-conditions/obesity/handling-the-psychological-and-emotional-effects-of-dramatic-weight-loss

97. https://www.mymed.com/diseases-conditions/obesity/handling-the-psychological-and-emotional-effects-of-dramatic-weight-loss

98. https://www.healthline.com/nutrition/maintain-weight-loss#TOC_TITLE_HDR_12

99. https://www.goodhousekeeping.com/health/diet-nutrition/a35697710/good-bad-foods-no-such-thing/

100. https://www.healthline.com/nutrition/most-weight-loss-friendly-foods#18

101. https://mypositiveparenting.org/2015/02/15/bad-vs-good-eating-habits-among-children/

102. https://www.healthline.com/nutrition/best-diet-plans

103. https://www.healthline.com/nutrition/best-weight-loss-meal-plans-for-women#how-to-choose

104. https://www.eatright.org/food/planning-and-prep/smart-shopping/3-strategies-for-successful-meal-planning

105. Barbara Gordan, "3 Strategies for Successful Meal Planning", 2019

106. https://www.healthline.com/nutrition/weight-loss-diet-plan-for-men#10.-Vegetarian-diets

107. https://www.eatright.org/food/nutrition/dietary-guidelines-and-myplate/healthy-eating-for-women

108. https://www.mayoclinic.org/healthy-lifestyle/childrens-health/in-depth/nutrition-for-kids/art-20049335

109. https://www.who.int/news-room/fact-sheets/detail/healthy-diet

110. Han Carrel, Stop Smoking Easy, 2017 www.bookyourdestiny.com

Printed in Great Britain
by Amazon